GET ACCURATE ANSWERS TO ALL YOUR QUESTIONS ABOUT KNEE PAIN— AND AVOID UNNECESSARY SURGERY!

- I've been told that I have torn knee cartilage. Do I need surgery?
- My knee makes funny noises. Is that a problem?
- What is "knee arthritis"?
- Can an MRI tell me why my knee hurts?
- How do I choose the right physical therapy for my knee condition?
- Do nutritional supplements work for knee pain?
- Is it better to apply heat or cold to the knee?
- If I have arthritis, should I take calcium?
- How do I know when I really need surgery?
- Which different operations should I know about?

Don't take chances with your knees! Get concise, straightforward answers to these and dozens of other questions, plus expert medical advice and proven exercises for relieving nagging knee pain—*without surgery*—in Dr. Ronald P. Grelsamer's . . .

WHAT YOUR DOCTOR MAY *NOT* TELL YOU ABOUT KNEE PAIN AND SURGERY

what your doctor may *not* tell you about
KNEE PAIN
— and —
SURGERY

Learn the Truth about MRIs and Common Misdiagnoses—and Avoid Unnecessary Surgery

Ronald P. Grelsamer, M.D.

WARNER BOOKS

An AOL Time Warner Company

Warner Books, Inc., 1271 Avenue of the Americas, New York, NY 10020

Visit our Web site at www.twbookmark.com.

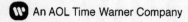 An AOL Time Warner Company

The title of the series What Your Doctor May *Not* Tell You About . . . and the related trade dress are trademarks owned by Warner Books, Inc., and may not be used without permission.

Printed in the United States of America

First Printing: February 2002

10 9 8 7 6 5 4 3 2 1

ISBN: 0-446-67819-8
LCCN: 2001096743

Book design by Charles S. Sutherland
Cover design by Brigid Pearson
Cover photo by Roseanne Olson/Stone

To my wife, Sharon, whose patience has made this book possible, and to Dr. Frank Stinchfield who taught me to treat each patient like a friend.

ACKNOWLEDGMENTS

I was absent during many a family outing to complete this book, and for Sharon, Dominique, and Marc's tolerance I will be eternally grateful.

I also wish to thank my professors at Columbia University's New York Orthopaedic Hospital for having instilled in me the basic values of medical care. Special thanks to Drs. Frank Stinchfield, Hugo Keim, Jean-Pierre Farcy, Nas Eftekhar, Charles Neer III, David Andrews, Louis Bigliani, Mel Rosenwasser, Roslyn Kane, Harold Dick, S. Ashby Grantham, Marvin Shelton, David Roye, Robert Carroll, Stephen McIlveen, Christopher Michelson, CAL Bassett, Shearwood McClelland, Austin Johnson, and May Parisien. With the passage of time their sense of ethics appears even more admirable.

Perhaps the best medical advice I ever received was the admonition of Dr. Frank Stinchfield to greet all patients as though I'd been waiting all day to see them and to dispense advice as if each were a friend.

Many thanks to my agent, Ms. Gareth Esersky, for steering me into the capable hands of Mr. John Aherne, Ms. Penina Sacks, and their wonderful team at Warner Books. The little 20,000-word treatise has gradually grown into the all-inclusive, sixteen-chapter text you are now holding!

CONTENTS

Chapter 1

Why Doctors Misinform You

DOCTORS ARE EARNEST AND INTELLIGENT, ARE BLESSED WITH an excellent memory, and are dedicated to making people feel better. For the most part.

Alas, there also exists a being I call the *LK-SS (Limited Knowledge–Suspect Scruples) doctor.* This is the kind of doctor you have to watch out for.

LIMITED KNOWLEDGE

It seems incredible that after four years of medical school and four to six more years of orthopedic training, an orthopedist or physiatrist (rehabilitation specialist) could still be deficient in his or her knowledge of the knee. And yet it's true. Over the last four decades, the world of orthopedics has become huge.

When I was in training in the early 1980s, some of my

teachers had had no formal training in orthopedic surgery (i.e., the surgery of bones and joints). They had trained as general surgeons and somewhere along the line had taken an interest in orthopedics. Up until the 1960s the sum total of orthopedic knowledge was small enough that any general surgeon could indulge in orthopedic surgery. General surgeons, for example, routinely set fractured bones.

Then the field became more sophisticated. A different approach was developed for every type of fracture in each bone. Moreover, for each of these fractures, controversies developed. The world of fractures became a field unto itself that could no longer be considered a small surgical aside. Techniques were also perfected for spinal deformities, arthritis, sports trauma, and pediatric conditions. Such operations were too numerous for a general surgeon to simply handle in his spare time. By the 1980s, surgeons who had taken specialty training in orthopedic surgery were addressing most of the orthopedic conditions treated in the United States.

Incredibly, orthopedics became yet more complicated. Each part of the body became a specialty unto itself. Consider the scientific literature: There are at least two English-language journals dealing only with knees, many journals dealing only with sports injuries, and entire journals devoted to *only* the hand, shoulder, spine, foot, joint replacements, fractures, or children's orthopedics.

People were amazed in the 1970s when an entire book was devoted to the knee. Now even the knee is nearly too broad a subject. I have written a medical textbook dealing exclusively with the kneecap—and it's the third textbook on the subject!

A medical-school curriculum calls for, at the very most, one or two weeks of orthopedic training sandwiched in between "more important" subjects. With occasional exceptions, medical students know next to nothing about orthopedics when they graduate.

The LK-SS Doctor

- *Limited Knowledge:* Not every orthopedist, rehabilitation doctor, or physical therapist is expert in the knee!
- *Suspect Scruples:* For some doctors, it's very tempting to recommend surgery.

An orthopedist in training is already an M.D. and is called a resident. He or she learns the basics pertaining to each part of the body and how to perform the most common procedures. All orthopedists learn to recognize and treat fractures. However, the world of orthopedics is too vast for an orthopedist out of general training to know all there is to know about hands, feet, knees, shoulders, etc. So orthopedists often now do fellowships, and learn from one or two doctors whatever it is that those doctors specialize in. Thus, there are hand fellowships, spine fellowships, and so forth. There are very few knee fellowships. This is because for historical reasons the world of knee surgery has been split into two parts. Right from its onset, in the early to mid-1970s, knee-replacement surgery fell into the orbit of hip-replacement surgery, which had already existed for approximately a decade. Surgeons proficient in hip replacement surgery initially performed most of the knee replacements. On the other hand, knee arthroscopies and ligament reconstructions were first performed in the early 1980s by the sports orthopedists. Therefore, there exist joint-replacement surgeons and fellowships for knee arthritis and sports surgeons and fellowships for just about every other knee problem. We have an entire generation of orthopedists knowledgeable in only one aspect of the knee (sports surgery versus joint-replacement surgery), not to mention orthopedists in general who have never had a specific interest in knees to begin with.

If you have an obvious, common problem, any orthopedist will be able to give you good advice. (Whether he chooses to do so is another subject, as we will discuss below.) But the more subtle problems will go undiagnosed. Consequently, the doctor may resort to unnecessary expensive testing, "let's go in and see" surgery, and lengthy, unproductive sessions of unfocused physical therapy.

SUSPECT SCRUPLES

This is a delicate subject. As a practicing orthopedic surgeon, I am talking about my colleagues, people I work with and have helped train, people I see at every meeting who I hope will come to my courses and buy my textbooks. But let's face it. A number of orthopedists and physiatrists are not straightforward. They are a minority, but not a small one. Your odds of getting a dishonest opinion range from 10 to 50 percent, depending on the setting. Some of the less honest doctors are new to their practice and will do anything to get started in a competitive market; others are chairmen of departments who abuse their prestige. They work in small hospitals; they operate out of large university centers. They are friendly, smooth-talking, and persuasive. They work side-by-side with excellent, knowledgeable, trustworthy doctors from whom they are outwardly indistinguishable. (Read chapter 15 to tell them apart.)

There are shades of dishonesty. Sometimes the doctors are blatantly dishonest, as when they state that something is fine when they know it isn't (or vice versa). But there are more subtle forms of dishonesty: failing to correct a patient's misinformation and misunderstanding. For example, you might undergo a sophisticated test, such as an MRI, and the report will read "grade II tear" of the cartilage. You think, *Torn cartilage; I need surgery.* Not so. A grade II tear is really not a tear at all and requires no surgery. But the LK-SS surgeon will not tell you this and will happily allow you to sign the surgical consent form. To the LK-SS surgery is irresistible. What better scenario (for a surgeon) than a patient expecting it? The patient is unlikely to know that he or she would have done equally well with more conservative measures.

Here is another scenario: A person has a severe arthritic flare-up in his or her knee and consults a specialist. The pain is so bad that he or she will do anything, which includes agreeing to surgery. Every orthopedist knows that the flare-up will eventually quiet down, especially if it is one of the first painful attacks. But the LK-SS surgeon will gladly offer to eliminate the problem with a knee replacement (soon, before the pain wears off). Don't scoff. This is not an uncommon scenario.

It is also deceitful to send patients for physical therapy that is not tailored to their specific condition. While some conditions can improve with twenty minutes of heat packs and cycling on an exercise bicycle, many require a more personal approach. But by sending you for plain, impersonal, bare-boned physical therapy that won't help you, the surgeon can tell you that you "failed physical therapy" and that you therefore need surgery.

Which brings us to the "perfect crime": The surgeon picks a high-tech, outpatient procedure that is associated with a low complication rate and a speedy recovery. The procedure is performed on a patient who would eventually do well, anyway. (One has to hurry up before the patient gets better on his or her own.) When the patient does get better, the surgeon is credited with the recovery, and many more patients are referred to him. Everybody wins—except the people paying the bills, but who cares?

Even educated people get tricked into surgery. I can imagine going to the dentist with a toothache and having the dentist send me for an expensive test. If the test came back saying I had some kind of dental rot, it wouldn't dawn on me that perhaps every test on every patient shows dental rot and that my trusty dentist was using that test to sell me an unnecessary procedure. So I sympathize fully with people who've been sold a knee arthroscopy. Therefore, the existence of this book. Physiatrists and chiropractors are not immune to the LK-SS phenomenon, either: Whereas surgeons exploit gullible patients with respect to surgery, LK-SS physiatrists and chiropractors relish endless therapy sessions.

Interestingly, if you have a personal-injury case, your attorney may unwittingly play a role in your getting inappropriate advice and treatment. The chances are overwhelming that your lawyer doesn't know the subtleties of MRI reports. When he sees "cartilage tear," he will think, just like you, that the tear is the result of an injury. From a business point of view, he will not be displeased that you need surgery; it makes for a stronger legal case. Likewise, it makes for a stronger case if you are receiving ongoing physical therapy, as it demonstrates persistent symptoms and a need for prolonged care.

Faced with both a patient and a lawyer who expect surgery and prolonged physical therapy, the LK-SS surgeon and physiatrist find it irresistible to schedule an operation and lengthy therapy, though not necessarily in that order.

In the following chapters we will review what you can do to protect yourself against misinformation and painfully suboptimal treatment.

Chapter 2

The MRI Lie

- "The knee didn't feel right to Conrad," Coach Jim Fassel said. "His knee was clicking, and he couldn't go on it. I told them I want an MRI now."[1]
- In the hands of the wrong orthopedist, the MRI becomes a license to operate.
- Treat patients, not tests.

In the twenty or so years since its development, the MRI has gone from being a medical curiosity to a major myth. In fact, the accuracy of the MRI is arguably one of the greatest myths in the world of orthopedic medicine, fueled by quotes such as the one attributed to football coach Jim Fassel of the New York Giants. Its roots lie in the awesome power of MRI technology.

1. *New York Times,* September 9, 1999.

WHAT IS AN MRI?

MRI stands for magnetic resonance imaging. It is an extra-ordinary tool that allows doctors to look inside the human body. It consists of a narrow, flat table on which the patient rests. Patient and table are surrounded by a huge magnet. The MRI produces black-and-white pictures of the knee, shadows if you will (fig. 2.1). But, as groundbreaking as it is, the MRI creates nothing more than thin, flat slices of a complex, colorful three-dimensional structure. Imagine trying to re-create in your mind the shape of a funny-looking loaf of bread just by observing the slices on a plate. Therefore, MRIs are subject to interpretation. Doctors with varying degrees of experience and knowledge will read MRIs differently.

MRIS ARE IMPERFECT IN FOUR WAYS

MRIs can miss certain painful conditions:

• *Arthritis.* Arthritis has a specific textbook definition: the loss of articular cartilage, the shiny white material at the end of each bone. Arthritis can be confined to a small part of the knee or can involve the entire knee. If the arthritic area is small enough, it will not show up on an MRI—a common source of patient disappointment. When patients go to an orthopedist complaining of knee pain, they might be told that they have torn cartilage, they expect that an outpatient operation will fix it, and when they have persistent pain, the doctor explains that he found some arthritis. "How could that be? It didn't say so on the MRI!"

Caveat emptor! If you are over fifty years old and you have knee pain, you may well have an area of arthritis in your knee

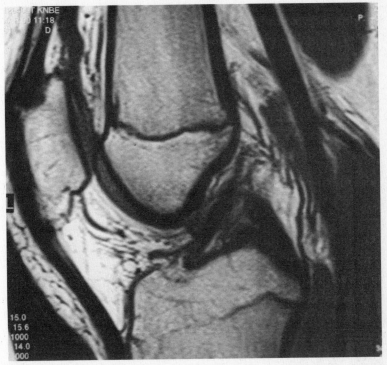

Fig. 2.1. A typical MRI picture of the knee (as seen on a side view).

that will *not* show up on an MRI. A competent doctor should explain this to you before you embark on any procedure.

• *Ligament tears.* Following a major injury, a completely shredded ligament will be detected on any MRI. However, an ACL (anterior cruciate ligament) that has been pulled off its attachment and has reattached itself to a neighboring structure may be read as normal. Indeed, the ligament still has a normal appearance; it has simply moved a half inch or so. A ligament that is painfully stretched can also be misread as normal.

Finally, an ACL that is partially torn—some of the fibers are normal, some are torn—will also appear normal on an MRI.

This is because the traditional MRI "slices" are 4 millimeters thick. Everything within those 4 millimeters is averaged. As long as there are enough healthy ligament fibers in any given slice, the MRI picture will appear normal. Imagine a thick slice of bread. Now imagine four rows of raisins in that slice. Even if you eliminate a whole row of raisins, your mouth will still taste "raisin bread." Even with three rows missing, it might taste like raisin bread. Had you cut the bread into thinner slices, your mouth might have noticed some missing raisins. Fortunately, a partially torn ligament can still function reasonably well (as can a loaf of bread with a few missing raisins). We'll discuss this further in chapter 4.

These Conditions May Be Missed on an MRI:

- early arthritis (chapter 5)
- partial ACL ligament tears (chapter 4)
- kneecap malalignment (chapter 6)
- bruising of skin and nerves (chapter 7)
- cartilage (meniscal tears)

• *Kneecap problems.* The kneecap (patella) can be poorly aligned in many different ways. Most of the time, the malalignment will be missed by the radiologist. In fact, a number of MRI centers do not even bother to take all the MRI cuts (views) necessary to judge the position of the kneecap. It saves money, and few people complain. The kneecap can "ride high"; in other words it can sit too far from the knee joint. The medical term for this is *patella alta,* which is a condition people can be born with, in which case it is said to be congenital; it can also be due to trauma. When the condition is traumatic, swelling and hemorrhage are present, and any radiologist can detect the abnormality. The congenital variety, however, is more subtle, and even if you're missing a few fingers, you can count on one hand the number of radiologists in this country who can diagnose a subtle high-riding kneecap. There are other forms of malalignment that are likely to be overlooked on an MRI. Which is a shame, because kneecap pain is quite common and difficult to treat. When you are trying to convince the insurance companies that you have a real problem, it doesn't make life easier to be holding an MRI report erroneously read as "normal."

• *Serious bruises of the skin and nerves.* If you strike your knee and painfully bruise your skin and the underlying nerves, the affected area will not be revealed on an MRI. Such conditions can result from having hit one's knees against the dashboard of a car, or from a fall.

• *Cartilage tears.* Between the femur (thighbone) and tibia (shinbone) lie two rubbery shock absorbers called the menisci (one meniscus; two menisci). Large tears can be picked up on an MRI, but smaller tears can go undetected. Remember: The MRI only shows you thin shadows of complex structures; therefore, small abnormalities can be missed. Small tears can still be quite painful and occasionally require surgery.

• *Any condition best detected with the patient in the standing position.* Because the MRI is performed on a subject who is lying down, conditions that are best observed with the patient in the standing position may be missed. These would include certain forms of arthritis and kneecap malalignment (see above).

At the other extreme, MRIs can overread conditions:

• *Torn cartilage.* The radiologist and orthopedist may feel that something is torn, and yet at surgery the structure is found to be intact. The reasons for this are complex and have to do

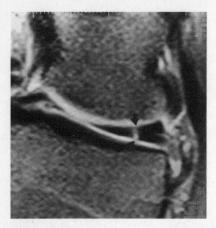

Fig. 2.2A. A true tear of the meniscus. Note how the white line goes all the way through the black. (The meniscus is black on an MRI.)

Fig. 2.2B. A phony tear. There is some white substance within the black, but the white line does not go all the way through. (Moreover, the white has been highlighted for this illustration.) This simply represents a chemical change within the meniscus, not a tear. Nevertheless, some radiologists would read this as a grade I tear, and the patient could be led to believe that he or she needs surgery.

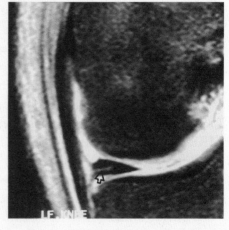

with "signal artifact." At this point I need to backtrack a little and review with you what a meniscus looks like on an MRI. A perfectly normal meniscus on an ideal MRI picture appears as a solid black triangle, somewhat akin to a baseball pennant (figs. 2.2 A & B). Occasionally, one finds a little blob of white in the middle of the triangle, just as there might be a slight flickering on your television screen. This little white blip is called an artifact, or signal change. (It can be due to the MRI hardware or software, or scarring from prior surgery. For example, a meniscus (fibrous cartilage) that has been operated on can still look torn on an MRI even if it is intact. This commonly leads to unnecessary repeat surgery.

> A radiologist can "create" the image of a torn cartilage by turning a knob on *his console!*

One of the most questionable practices in radiology is the reporting of normal signal changes in meniscal cartilage as tears (figs. 2.3 A & B). In the early days of MR imaging, these signal changes were graded from I to III. Grade I and II tears do not represent changes visible to the naked eye. Although some might argue that they represent tears at the microscopic level, they are certainly not tears that one could see or operate on.

Fig. 2.3A. A phony tear. The white within the black of the meniscus does not represent a clinically significant tear.

Fig. 2.3B. A true tear. The white band transects the meniscus.

I was most shocked a few years ago when a radiologist showed me how he could simply dial in a grade I or II tear by turning a knob on his MRI console!

It thus became easier for me to understand how certain radiologists might read a tear on every MRI. By reporting grade I and II changes as tears, the radiologist allows the unscrupulous orthopedic surgeon to "sell" the patient a surgical procedure: Seeing the word "tear" on the MRI report, most patients readily agree to surgery. In short, the MRI report has become a license to operate. The insurers don't know any better and readily approve the procedure. A grade III change, on the other hand, is more likely to represent a true tear. And even then there can be "false-positives," the scientific term for false alarm. It is the doctor's responsibility to correlate the test results with the patient's symptoms and physical examination. *A good doctor treats patients, not tests.*

These Conditions Will Be Overread by an MRI:

- torn cartilage (so common, it is nearly routine)
- a Baker's cyst
- tumors (rare)
- infection (rare)

• *A Baker's cyst.* In anticipation of a general outcry from my radiology colleagues, let me apologize ahead of time for including Baker's cysts in this section. Over a hundred years ago, Dr. Baker described a pouch of fluid commonly found at the back of the knee. The liquid is normal knee-joint fluid that in some people seeps through a small opening and collects in this pouch. The pouch varies in size from person to person. It ranges from being invisible to feeling like a large Ping-Pong ball. The swelling can come and go as the fluid moves back and forth from the cyst to the knee joint. *Unless the cyst is particularly large, it is usually asymptomatic and requires no treatment.* According to current thinking, fluid tends to build up in the knee—and thus into a Baker's cyst—when something is irritating the knee. That something can be any number of conditions, including arthritis or a true torn cartilage. The situation is analogous to tears in your eye. If something were to irritate your eye, it would tear. However, in the case of your eye, the tears escape down your cheek, whereas in the knee they have nowhere to go but into that Baker's cyst. The treatment of a Baker's cyst (which is rarely necessary) must therefore be focused on addressing the source of irritation within the knee (torn cartilage, arthritis, etc.). Occasionally, a one-way valve develops between the cyst and the knee: Fluid can get into the cyst but can't flow back to the joint. The body absorbs the fluid, but not completely: It leaves behind a jellylike substance that can actually harden with time. The doctor may place a needle in that cyst and aspirate (suck out) that substance. It may recur.

Most significantly, a Baker's cyst is readily seen on an MRI and is commonly listed on the MRI report. Radiologists are perfectly justified in listing it (thus, the above apology). The problem—and this is why I've included the Baker's cyst in this section—is that everyone but the patient understands that it is a common, harmless finding. Patients are understandably anxious at the thought of a cyst living around their knee. It is therefore not so much a question of an overread by the radiologist as an overinterpretation on the part of the patient. It doesn't help that in the radiologist's summation the innocent Baker's cyst is listed above the true culprit (e.g., arthritis; see page 16).

• *Bone tumors and infections.* An MRI is so sensitive that it detects the smallest change in tissue composition. Such changes occasionally give the appearance of a tumor or an infection, which is quite frightening. Fortunately, a biopsy will reveal the tissue to be normal.

The MRI does not tell you what hurts!

It is common for people to have an "abnormality" that is completely asymptomatic (pain-free). The mere presence of an abnormality does not signify that there is a problem that must be treated, and it is the doctor who must decide whether the so-called abnormality is truly the source of the problem. I have seen countless patients who have had MRI "abnormalities" surgically corrected and who still complain of the same pain. For example, I once treated a patient with knee pain who had had surgery for a torn cartilage. His MRI had clearly suggested a torn cartilage, but he still had pain despite the surgery. A further workup revealed that his knee pain was actually caused by a hip condition. The knee pain completely resolved once the hip was surgically repaired. This is by no means a rare scenario. The finding of a torn cartilage on an MRI is quite common, but it does not automatically tell you what hurts.

Some LK-SS orthopedists routinely dictate "MRI-confirmed meniscal tear" in their operative reports when describing the cartilage they have just "operated" on. This way, presumably, if the patient still has pain after surgery because the tear never existed or because it wasn't the source of the pain to begin with, the surgeon can blame the MRI. "It's not my fault, Mrs. Jones, that we chose the wrong operation. That MRI report did report torn cartilage, did it not?"

The MRI reports often emphasize the wrong condition.

An MRI report commonly reads something like this:

- tear of the meniscus
- water in the knee
- partial tear of such and such ligament
- Baker's cyst
- arthritis

While this report may technically be correct, the order of the conditions listed implies that the torn meniscus is the main problem. In most patients, however, the presence of arthritis supersedes all other afflictions. The patient will not improve until the arthritis is addressed, whereas little tears of the meniscus, water in the knee, and partial tears of ligaments are not likely to be the source of the patient's pain. The bit about the "tear of the meniscus" does succeed in catching the eye of the patient and the unsuspecting family doctor, and it paves the way for an offer from the orthopedist to fix that nasty little problem with a surgical procedure.

ALL MRIS ARE NOT EQUIVALENT

You would be appalled by the variations in image quality from one MRI to another and by the differences in accuracy from one report to another. This is a reflection of the diversity among the four elements that make up an MRI and its accompanying report.

The MRI test has four components: the hardware (the machine), the software (the computer program that runs the machine), the radiologist, and the orthopedist (the type of doctor most likely to be looking at your knee).

The hardware

As with cars and planes, MRIs come in different models. The most obvious difference between them is their open versus closed nature. The closed models are tunnels into which a person is slid into via a narrow table. The open models are open on the sides. By and large, the closed models are more precise, but for many purposes the open ones will suffice. The main advantage of the open models lies in the diminished claustrophobia. Having said this, modern medications can dispel this claustrophobia, and a small Valium-like tablet can nearly turn a closed

MRI session into a relaxing experience. (Valium itself is not used because it lasts too long.)

The Variable Ingredients of an MRI:

- the machine
- the computer software
- the radiologist (who writes the report)
- the orthopedist (who reviews the MRI pictures and correlates them with your symptoms—or should!)

The software

As it does in any computer the software runs the hardware, and it is as important as the machine itself, which explains why the most beautiful MRI images do not necessarily come from the very latest machines. Understandably, the information pertaining to the software and to the hardware is not something readily available to the lay or orthopedic community.

The radiologist

This person is vastly underestimated. The radiologist can manipulate the software to highlight certain features of the knee. Two radiologists using the same machine can obtain different results! The radiologist has to interpret ("read") the pictures. Not all radiologists are equally adept at appreciating the subtleties of a knee MRI. What looks essentially normal to one radiologist can look somewhat irregular, swollen, displaced, or degenerated to another. What one radiologist reads as a tear, another reads as a simple *signal change* (radiology jargon for medically insignificant white or black spot on a magnetic image). Don't be fooled by the term *board certified* under a radiologist's name. Board certification doesn't make him or her an expert in every area of radiology. I am board certified in orthopedic surgery, but you wouldn't want me to operate on your spine!

Remember also that no radiologist can tell you what hurts.

The orthopedist

This is the person who should be correlating the MRI images with your symptoms. Some doctors simply scan the radiologist's report and read you the alleged diagnosis. This is a major mistake for the reasons listed above.

Note that the best orthopedist and the best radiologist can still disagree as to whether there is a cartilage or ligament tear or not or on whether the kneecap is normal or not. You would think that a radiologist would be more knowledgeable than an orthopedist when it comes to reading X rays and MRIs, and sometimes this is true. In certain cases, however, it is the reverse. The buck stops with the clinician looking after you. If an MRI is necessary to make the diagnosis, he (or she) must review the films himself.

The lawyers, insurance companies, and patients (the LIPs of the world) collectively and individually represent very powerful groups. As of this writing, LIPs assume that MRIs are perfect. They assume that anything that is wrong will show up on an MRI, they rely on the MRI report as if it came from a higher power, and they readily accept the concept that any abnormality on the MRI is painful and needs to be fixed. As we have seen above, nothing could be further from the truth. This attitude, however, plays directly into the hands of LK-SS orthopedists, and it completely skewers insurance and legal payouts (see chapters 12 and 13). Patients with painful conditions that are not apparent to the radiologist are denied coverage and compensation, while people with fictitious tears can be given significant rewards.

Chapter 3

"Life-Threatening" Torn Cartilage

*B*AD NEWS: THERE'S A GOOD CHANCE THAT AN MRI WILL show that you have torn cartilage in your knee.

More bad news: If this report lands in the hands of an LK-SS orthopedist (see chapter 1) you will be told that you need surgery.

Good news: He's pulling your leg. Chances are that you don't need surgery.

At the dawn of this new millennium, you are at greater risk of being misdiagnosed with a torn cartilage *than at any other time in history.* Once upon a time, surgery for a torn cartilage required one or two big incisions about the knee. Surgeons thought twice about performing this kind of surgery. No more.

Now that the procedure is "minor," unscrupulous surgeons perform them at a remarkable clip.

WHAT IS A "TORN CARTILAGE"?

The medical profession is responsible for having coined one term for two very different structures: Cartilage is the name given to the smooth white material that lines the end of bone. (Check it out the next time you eat chicken.) Although never "torn," cartilage may wear out. The wearing-out process is called arthritis.

> ## Cartilage Is Both:
>
> • the shiny white material at the end of a bone and
> • the rubbery shock absorbers inside the knee.

Cartilage is also the colloquial name given to the thin, rubbery shock absorbers inside the knee between the thighbone (femur) and shinbone (tibia) known in the medical world as the menisci ("men-IS-kai." One meniscus, two menisci) (fig. 3.1). These structures can be torn; therefore, the term *torn cartilage.*

Menisci are crescent-shaped, and there are two in each knee—one toward the inner part of the knee (medial) and the other toward the outside (lateral). By virtue of their somewhat crescent/cupped shape, they add stability to the knee. In other words, they help keep the knees from being wobbly. Because of their cushy nature, they also provide shock absorption.

When the doctor says, "You have torn cartilage," he is referring to one (or both) of those menisci.

How Does a Cartilage Tear?

A (meniscal) cartilage tears in one of two ways:

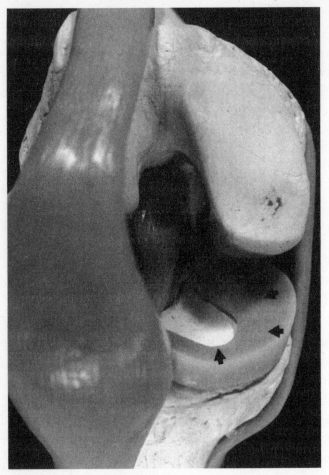

Fig. 3.1. The meniscus is a rubbery, crescent-shaped shock absorber. It rests on the surface of the shinbone (black arrows). There are two in each knee.

1. A sudden injury. You get up from a seated position on the floor, feel a pop, and can't straighten the knee. Chances are you tore a meniscus.

2. Wear and tear. Most tears fall into this category. The natu-

ral aging process causes chemical changes in the meniscus, more so in some people than in others. These changes in turn predispose the meniscus to fraying and tearing. The posterior (toward the back of the knee) aspect of the meniscus is subject to higher stresses than the rest of the meniscus, and recent research suggests that the back of the meniscus is also mechanically weaker. Not surprisingly, then, it is the most likely part of the meniscus to tear.

What Does a Torn Cartilage Feel Like?

The pain is usually localized in one specific part of the knee. You can just about put your finger on it. With the knee bent at a right angle, as when sitting in a chair, the tenderness is typically right between the thighbone and the shinbone, the so-called joint line. Bending down is particularly painful. When there is a large bucket-handle tear (see fig. 3.2 D), you can't completely straighten out the knee (but keep in mind that even minor ligament injuries can also do this for a few days after the trauma; see chapter 4).

What Other Conditions Feel Like a Torn Cartilage?

There are many causes of knee pain. If you are between the ages of twenty and forty, you may simply have a nagging tendinitis, an inflammation of a tendon. You may have a subtle problem with your kneecap (chapter 6). You may have "runner's knee," an irritation of the so-called iliotibial band, which runs along the outside of the leg and knee (chapter 7).

The MRI report may indicate torn cartilage, but the real cause of your pain may be one of the conditions listed above. As noted repeatedly in this book, many people without knee pain appear to have a torn cartilage, as seen on an MRI. Therefore, the mere presence of such a torn cartilage does not indicate the source of a person's pain.

> Not all cartilage tears are painful!

What Does a Torn Cartilage Look Like?

A meniscus can tear in an infinite variety of ways: There are so-called bucket-handle, parrot-beak, radial, cleavage, flap, degenerative tears, and every permutation thereof (figs. 3.2 A–E). A bucket-handle tear is very large and involves a major portion of the meniscus. The others are usually localized in the back of the meniscus. The back and front portions of the meniscus are called *horns*. Therefore, a common finding on an MRI report is "a tear of the posterior horn of the medial meniscus."

Are All Tears Equivalent?

No. Many radiologists continue to grade tears into categories I, II, and III. Grade I and II tears represent chemical changes or scratches not visible to the naked eye. A grade III tear represents a through-and-through tear that is clearly visible.

This is a critical difference. A grade III tear may or may not require surgery. A grade I or II tear never does! Every orthopedic surgeon knows this. The LK-SS surgeon, however, routinely counts on your ignorance to sell you an operation for a grade I or II tear.

That lawyers are not aware of the difference—neither your lawyer nor those of the insurance companies—can work for or against you. Usually this works in your favor, since a "torn cartilage" of any kind is assumed to represent a significant injury.

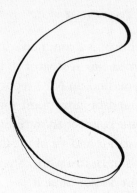

Fig. 3.2A. Normal meniscus.

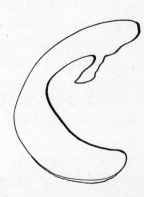

Fig. 3.2B. Flap tear of meniscus.

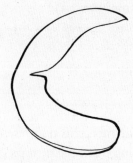

Fig. 3.2C. Radial tear of meniscus.

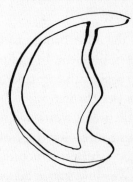

Fig. 3.2D. "Bucket-handle" tear of meniscus.

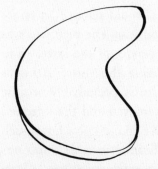

Fig. 3.2E. Discoid meniscus. It is thicker than the normal meniscus and closer to looking like a disc.

Can You Get Arthritis from a Torn Cartilage?

"Let's take care of this before you get arthritis" is a common scare tactic to get you to surgery. Nonsense medicine is what it is. In the first place, the common tears that you find on MRI reports will not cause arthritis: As you understand by now, most torn cartilages found on MRI reports have little connection to reality. By and large, true tears occur in older patients and are of the degenerative, that is, wear-and-tear, type—similar to a worn carpet. They may be associated with arthritis but do not cause it.

Scare Tactic

"If we don't operate on this tear, you'll get arthritis."

On the other hand, major tears of the meniscus do present a potential problem. In addition to causing pain, the torn piece can rub against the articular cartilage, wear it down, and cause arthritis (see chapter 5).

Until twenty years ago, surgeons would remove an entire meniscus to treat any type of meniscal tear. The meniscus was felt to be a useless structure, the appendix of the knee, so to speak. We now know better. Removing the entire meniscus greatly increases a person's risk of arthritis, presumably because the knee's shock absorber has been removed and the knee has been rendered somewhat less stable. We do not know how much meniscus has to be removed to significantly increase someone's risk for arthritis. Nowadays, surgeons therefore remove as little meniscus as possible—the torn portion, no more, no less. A partial meniscectomy is performed.

The younger the patient, the less the surgeon removes. If arthritis develops in an older patient, there is always the option of a knee replacement. That option is not as palatable in the younger patient (see chapter 5). In fact, there is no great option when treating arthritis in the younger patient. The best treatment is therefore prevention, and prevention in this case means leaving as much of the meniscus as possible.

Do Even Educated People Get Tricked into Surgery?

You bet. As noted in chapter 1, educated or not, you tend to trust your doctor.

THE PHYSICAL EXAMINATION

In the days before MRIs, your doctor would make the diagnosis of a torn meniscus by listening to your story (the history) and by examining your knee. You can still make a strong case for the following point of view: A significant tear of the meniscus is best diagnosed during the physical examination.

If the tear is very large as in, say, a bucket-handle tear (see fig. 3.2 D), the torn piece will interfere with the mechanics of the knee. The knee will lock up. It's as if you stuck your finger in some big machine. *The knee won't straighten or will refuse to bend.* You will feel a mechanical stop. The knee will bend and straighten freely until it reaches a certain point. It will then seem to be blocked as if by a doorstop. The doctor then has his first clue. Mind you, it takes a *very* big tear to cause such locking. Conversely, there is hardly anything else that can cause such predictable and reproducible locking. You could argue convincingly that an MRI is unnecessary in this setting.

> In a true locked knee, the knee won't straighten all the way, as if stuck by a doorstop.

The meniscus lives between the thighbone and shinbone in a space that is easy to palpate when the knee is bent. This space is called the joint space. When a meniscus is torn, the tissues around it become inflamed. An analogy can be made here with a hangnail. In fact, in many ways, a torn meniscus is a hangnail of the knee. The inflammation around the torn meniscus causes pain, and *when the doctor presses his finger against the joint space, it hurts!* This finding is present with just about any significant tear. It is also found in the presence of arthritis and is therefore not specific to a meniscal tear. Nevertheless, it provides yet another clue for the doctor. In a patient not likely to have arthritis, namely someone under forty, it is an even bigger clue.

> Some time-honored tests are not very useful.

A classic test for a torn meniscus is the *McMurray test.* The patient lies on his or her back. The knee is bent. The doctor straightens the knee while turning the foot. If a dull clunk is perceived, the test is considered positive for a torn meniscus. I don't rely on this test because it is too inaccurate: You can have a painfully torn meniscus without having a positive McMurray test, and a positive McMurray test does not automatically indicate the presence of a significant tear. The following story illustrates the point: Frank Stinchfield, M.D., at one time the preeminent orthopedist in the United States and the teller of this story, went to visit Dr. McMurray in Great Britain. Mc-

Murray had just published his McMurray test and was eager to demonstrate it. "Lie down, Frank" he said, "and I'll show you how it's done." Dr. Stinchfield hiked himself up onto the examination table and bared his knee. McMurray performed his test, and they both heard a dull pop. "Why Frank, you have a torn meniscus!" "Amazing," replied Dr. Stinchfield. "My knee doesn't even hurt. Let me try it on you." With that he trades places with McMurray and performs the test on him. They both hear a clunk. "Wow," says Dr. Stinchfield. "You have a tear, too!" "Nonsense," snapped McMurray, with which he walked out in a huff. So much for the McMurray test. Nevertheless, the occasional insurance doctor will say, "And did your doctor perform a McMurray test?" as if it mattered.

Another test is the *Apley grind.* Here the patient lies on his or her stomach, with the knee bent at a right angle. The doctor pushes on the heel and twists the leg as if to grind the knee into the examination table. The idea is to perform a little Watusi on the torn meniscus and elicit pain. The problem here is that unless the patient is quite small and slender, it is difficult for the doctor to simulate with his arm the forces generated by the patient when he or she carries out the normal activities of daily living.

DO YOU NEED SURGERY FOR A TORN CARTILAGE?

A. Yes, you do need surgery if your knee pain is clearly the result of a tear *and* the pain interferes significantly with your everyday activities. Believe it or not, it is not always easy to determine at first glance whether torn cartilage is or is not the source of your pain.

First of all, the torn cartilage seen on the MRI may not be a tear at all. Little changes that are of no consequence are routinely read as cartilage tears (see chapter 2). What's worse, these little changes can be introduced by the radiologist simply by the turn of a dial. These so-called false-positive tears are the knee equivalent of a false alarm.

> An unscrupulous radiologist can "create" a torn carti- lage by turning a dial on his console.

In my experience, the odds of coming across a false-positive MRI range from 10 to 100 percent, depending on the knowl- edge and integrity of the radiologist. Since a reading of torn meniscus presents the unscrupulous orthopedist with a license to operate, an equally unscrupulous radiologist reads a torn meniscus in essentially everyone. This ensures him continued business from the orthopedist and lawyer, if there is one who is part of the "Game" (see chapter 13).

Moreover, not all tears are painful. The knowledgeable ortho- pedist will carefully examine other parts of the knee before pro- nouncing the meniscus the likely source of pain. The LK-SS, alas, will pounce on the MRI report and announce that he has found the source of your pain without ever looking for any other cause.

Finally, some tears will not be visible on an MRI. They may be small or subtle. Nevertheless, they can be a source of pain. A normal MRI therefore does not rule out a torn meniscus.

The torn cartilage can be a nuisance because it is painful or because it causes locking of the knee. Locking is the term used when the knee won't straighten because something is blocking it. That "something" is the piece of cartilage interfering with the intricate machinery of the knee. Again, the consumer must be- ware: There is so-called pseudolocking, where a knee won't straighten or bend simply because it hurts too much to do so.

The knowledgeable orthopedists can tell the difference. The LK-SS will use the pseudolocking to, once again, sell an operation. "Mrs. Smith, your knee is locked. We better get to this quickly."

B. No, you do *not* need surgery unless your knee pain is most likely the result of a tear *and* the pain interferes significantly with your activities of daily living.

> Not all torn cartilage requires surgery.

If You Do Need Surgery, Is It an Emergency?

Never. There is no such thing as life-threatening torn cartilage.

The LK-SS surgeon takes the shoe-salesman approach (no offense meant to shoe salesmen): Make the sale today or lose the customer. This may be reasonable in the retail world; it is downright unethical in dealing with a possible torn cartilage. Unless the knee is locked, cartilage surgery can always wait—and even then, it need not be done that day. Don't let yourself get pressured into signing on the dotted line.

THE "MIRACLE" OF MICROSURGERY AND LASER SURGERY

In keeping with the tone of this book, I am pulling your leg a little: There is no microsurgery for torn cartilage, and there is no miracle of laser surgery.

These terms, however, are commonly used by doctors to dazzle you and to liposuck the common sense out of your head. Microsurgery has a very specific meaning in the world of surgery: surgery performed with the use of an operating-room microscope. When severed tendons, ligaments, and blood vessels are reattached, the surgeon not uncommonly resorts to microsurgery. No microscope is used in cartilage surgery, therefore, there is no microsurgery.

The term *laser* is an acronym for light amplification by stimulated emission of radiation, not, as some cynics would have it, limited applications of sophisticated and expensive research. In conventional arthroscopic surgery, the orthopedist employs miniaturized instruments to snip away at torn tissue. With lasers, the surgeon heats the tissue until it is vaporized. The end result is the same. I myself operated with an advanced holmium laser for six months. I presented a study at the American Society for Lasers in Medicine and Surgery. I also taught laser safety for a major medical-laser manufacturer. The point is that, if anything, I am partial to lasers. Having said this, the advantage of a laser in the setting of a torn cartilage is limited.[1] A laser does not speed up the surgery, improve recovery, or diminish the risks of surgery. If a surgeon tries to impress you with the use of a laser, you know you are dealing with an LK-SS. As of this writing, lasers in knee surgery are mainly used as a marketing tool. Many patients are impressed at the thought of having a laser procedure. The doctors and hospitals know this.

The True Miracle

Because cartilage surgery is performed so frequently, it is easy to lose sight of the fact that it does represent a small miracle of technology. The procedure used to address torn cartilage is called an arthroscopy (ar-THROS-cup-ee) from the Greek

1. R. P. Grelsamer, "Should Lasers Be Used in Orthopedic Surgery?" *Orthopedic Special Edition* 3, no. 1 (1997): 49.

arthro (joint) and *scop* (to look). A slender pencil-like tube is introduced into the knee. The tube is connected to a palm-sized camera that is connected to a television monitor. Thus, the inside of your knee is projected onto the television screen.

Note that nowhere in the word *arthroscopy* does the word *knee* appear. Indeed, an arthroscopy can be performed on any joint. A "scope" can be performed in any bodily cavity: cystoscopy (bladder), fundoscopy (uterus), laparoscopy (abdomen), to name but a few.

There Are Four Types of Anesthesia:

- general
- spinal (or epidural)
- local
- LMA

Through a separate puncture hole, tiny instruments are introduced. These instruments are long, slender rods at the end of which are miniaturized scissors, clippers, and shavers. They come in a multitude of shapes designed to reach the various nooks and crannies inside the knee.

Although most patients do not want to hear or see anything, it is possible for the person undergoing the procedure to observe the surgery on the same TV screen that is being watched by the surgeon. (You may not be allowed to wear your glasses or contact lenses!)

One chooses between four anesthetics:

1. *General intubation,* whereby you are put to sleep via an intravenous medication, and your respiration is assured via a plastic tube gently slipped down your windpipe. With just the

right amount of intravenous medication, it is possible to wake up rather quickly and be on your way home in just a few hours.

2. A *spinal or epidural.* A local anesthetic is injected into your lower back. This is below your spinal cord, and as such, paralysis is not a realistic complication. With this approach, you can remain wide awake if you so desire, or you can receive intravenous sedation, which "knocks you out," though not as deeply as with general anesthesia. It may take a few hours for the spinal to wear off; in the meantime, you must stay in the recovery room.

3. *Local anesthetic.* A Novocain type of medication is injected directly into the knee. In my experience, this is the least reliable type of anesthesia. Because there are many nooks and crannies in the knee, the medication may not reach each and every spot. The person opting for this has to be willing to accept the possibility of some pain and understand that he or she may require some intravenous sedation. How long one stays in the recovery room after a local depends strictly on how much added sedation was given during the surgery.

4. A variation of general and local is the use of a *rubber diaphragm "LMA"* (laryngeal-mask airway), which is placed in the back of the throat and connected to a ventilator—essentially general anesthesia without a tube down the windpipe. Depending on which anesthesiologist you speak to, this technique combines either the best or the worst of both worlds.

In my experience, these options are all approximately equal except for the local anesthetic, for the reasons listed above. If the anesthesiologist has a strong preference for one approach or the other, I tend to go with that approach. The anesthesiologist is one person I hate to upset.

WHAT IS BAND-AID SURGERY?

Band-Aid surgery is the same as minor surgery: surgery on somebody else. The terms Band-Aid surgery and minor surgery are used to impress upon you that the procedure will be quick, painless, and risk-free. You won't need a surgical dressing, just a Band-Aid. This is relatively true. The procedure itself is quick, but there can be a day and a half of pain thereafter. The chance of getting a significant complication is low but not zero. Infections, though rare, can occur. They lead to a significant amount of pain, further surgery, and a long course of antibiotics, which may need to be administered intravenously. Some patients develop severe stiffness; still others develop a painful condition called reflex sympathetic dystrophy (RSD), whereby pain fibers refuse to shut down and continue to send painful signals to the brain. As for just using a Band-Aid, some people can get a fair amount of oozing for a day or so after surgery, and it is simply not appropriate to employ such a small bandage.

> Band-Aid and minor surgery: surgery on somebody else!

RECOVERY AND REHABILITATION

Do you need physical therapy? When do you go back to work?

The beauty of performing cartilage surgery through two or three small puncture holes is that the *recovery* is infinitely faster than surgery carried out through a long skin incision. If you can be driven to work and if your work is sedentary, you can be back to work in three days. If you take a bus or subway or if you must stand on your feet a great deal, ten days is a more reasonable time to take off. Keep in mind that everyone is different. Resist the temptation to compare yourself to someone else. In some cases, for example, the knee has to be gently twisted during surgery for the surgeon to gain access to the torn cartilage, and this can prolong the recovery.

I find that approximately 50 percent of patients need physical therapy. People who, within a few days of surgery, still have trouble straightening the knee or bending it to 90 degrees are good candidates for formal physical therapy. Patients who find that their leg is wobbly and are not good at exercising on their own are also sent for physical therapy. Contrary to what we find with kneecap problems, therapy following arthroscopic cartilage surgery is reasonably standard: The therapist will apply heat and gently work on moving the knee. So-called modalities, such as ultrasound, can also be soothing. The therapist will stretch and massage the structures around the knee that have tightened up.

You Know You're Being Had When the Doctor

- examines your knee very briefly.
- says, "According to the MRI report, you have torn cartilage."
- announces that he can easily fix that for you.

Can I exercise on my own after surgery?

If you have the discipline, the answer is absolutely yes. You may want one session of physical therapy to verify that you are performing the exercises correctly, but then you can certainly be on your own.

First, you want to make sure that your knee straightens all the way. (A painful knee wants to stay slightly bent.) Sit on the floor or a firm mattress with the leg out straight and work on getting the back of the knee up against that surface. Hold the muscles tight for about ten seconds. Count to three and start again. Do this five to ten minutes at a time. It will seem like an eternity. I recommend music or television to fight the boredom.

At the opposite extreme, you want the knee to *bend*. The knee will be puffy from the fluid that was pumped through during the surgery, but you should be able to flex to 90 degrees (a right angle) within a few days. Sit on a table or bar stool, support your leg with the top of the other foot, and gradually let the knee bend.

It's amazing how quickly muscles become weak. Both fluid in the knee and pain can lead to muscle atrophy in the blink of an eye. Fortunately, this is easily reversible. Once you've regained reasonable motion in the knee—straightening it all the way and bending it 90 degrees—you can begin to strengthen it. Start with the classic straight-leg raise. Lie down and, without bending the knee, lift the heel an inch or so off the ground. Hold it off the ground for about ten seconds. Count to three and repeat. Continue five to ten minutes at a time. It's as boring as it is effective (see above). When this becomes too easy, attach a light weight to the ankle (one pound) and repeat. The lower leg acts as a long lever arm, so one pound at the ankle is more impressive than it sounds, especially on a painful knee. You can then progress in one-to-two-pound increments. You'll know when you're pretty much back to where you were before surgery.

Leg extensions are another classic exercise whereby you sit on a table or bar stool and gradually straighten the knee. I recommend starting with a one-pound weight at the ankle and then gradually working up to heavier weights. Again, remember: The lower leg is a long lever. The effect of the weight on your ankle gets multiplied by the length of this lever. Go easy on weight increases. One-to-two-pound increases are reasonable.

Are there exercises to avoid? Absolutely. Wall slides are one example. For this exercise, you place your back flush against the wall and gradually assume a sitting position. The farther away your feet are from the wall, the harder it is. It's a fine exercise for people with good knees looking to get stronger legs. It puts terrific stress on your kneecaps, though, and for many people it is painful. Try it if you want, but don't persist if it's the least bit painful. Which brings us to the next point: no pain, no gain.

This is a common adage. When a joint is stiff, it is reasonable to expect some discomfort, since it is being stretched. But *no* strengthening exercise should be painful. If it is, back off on the weights or stop altogether.

Is pool therapy recommended?

Absolutely. People with pools barely need physical therapy after an arthroscopy. Being buoyant makes it easier to stand on the leg. Moving the leg in the water provides natural resistance. Kicking in the water (any style) is a solid strengthening exercise. (Ever see swimmers' legs?) Lakes work well, too, although water that is too cold can make you tense up. I do not care for oceans if there are any waves or sudden drop-offs, which are too dangerous. You need a warm, controlled environment. (Try a trip to the Caribbean. Medicare and HMOs routinely cover that.)

When can I get my leg wet after surgery?

Within a few days, the puncture holes are reasonably sealed. Therefore, as soon as the dressing is off, I allow patients to shower. Water might still theoretically seep in if the leg is soaked in water; because of this, I do not allow bathing or swimming until ten days or so after surgery.

Moist heat or dry heat?

Even though they are opposites, heat and cold can both be soothing. For straightforward exercises, the traditional approach is to "warm up, ice down." Massage the knee and apply heat, in any form, prior to exercise. Five minutes should be fine. At the end of the exercise, apply a cold pack.

If you are looking to control pain, I would alternate heat and cold every five to ten minutes until you find the one that is best for you. I would then use whichever you've chosen for as much of the day as is practical for you.

For Pain Relief

Moist heat? Dry heat? Cold? Ice?
Whatever works for you.

Trick of the Trade

Rather than hold the heat or cold pack in your hands, wrap an elastic bandage (e.g., Ace) once or twice around the knee. Then apply the cold/heat pack. Finish wrapping the bandage. The cold/heat pack will stay in place. There are also some commercially available neoprene wraps that will do this for you in an even more convenient manner.

Heat can be dry, as when a heating pad is used, or moist, when a hot towel or electric hydrocollator is used. From a medical point of view, both are acceptable. You should use the form that works best for you.

UNUSUAL CONDITIONS

A small percentage of the population walks around with a so-called *discoid meniscus.* This is a meniscus that looks like a poker chip rather than a crescent. Discoid menisci come in different flavors: an incomplete discoid meniscus has an opening in the middle. The opening can be small or large. An incomplete discoid meniscus therefore can come close to looking like a normal meniscus or, at the other extreme, can essentially look like the traditional, complete discoid variety. The discoid meniscus can have normal peripheral attachments to the knee or can be completely detached from the back of the knee (the Wrisberg type of discoid meniscus). A Wrisberg discoid meniscus can cause snapping that eventually becomes painful. Surgery is required. It is challenging surgery because the meniscus has never been normally attached to the knee. There are no natural connections between the discoid meniscus and the knee capsule; in fact, the meniscus can be quite a distance from where it should be. This is a very different scenario from that of a normal meniscus that becomes detached and needs to be reattached.

The treatment of a discoid meniscus consists of removing part of the meniscus (a partial meniscectomy). As usual, the surgeon will try to remove as little as possible for fear of predisposing his patient to early arthritis. On the other hand, because the meniscus can be so abnormal, it may require nearly total removal before the patient becomes asymptomatic (pain-free). One has to hope that by the time our young patients develop arthritis, we will have even more treatment options than we have today.

Chapter 4

Stamp Out Torn Ligaments

C*ASE 1:* JANE IS SKIING IN SOFT SNOW WHEN SUDDENLY SHE catches the tip of her ski and feels a sharp pain in the left knee. The doctor says that she needs an MRI and ligament reconstruction—soon.

Case 2: Bill lands awkwardly from a jump and feels a painful pop in the right knee. The doctor informs him that he has a "torn ACL" and needs surgery—tomorrow.

Is this good advice?

A ligament is a sophisticated biological rope connecting two bones.[1] Some joints are quite solid (stable), and the ligaments are somewhat expendable. The hip joint, which consists of a large ball in a deep socket, is an example of such a joint. Even with a few ligaments removed, the hip ball does not come out of its socket. The knee and shoulder are at the other extreme.

---

1. A tendon links a *muscle* to a bone.

The knee can be likened to two large knobs resting on a flat surface. Without ligaments, this structure would be completely unstable. The thighbone would slide off the shinbone, as would a ball off the end of a table. In a patient this would translate to the knee giving out.

There are four ligaments in and about the knee (figs. 4.1, 2, & 4):

- the medial collateral ligament (MCL),
- the lateral (or fibular) collateral ligament (LCL),
- the posterior cruciate ligament (PCL), and
- the anterior cruciate ligament (ACL) (which the orthopedist most commonly gets to operate on).

The Four Ligaments of the Knee:

- MCL (most commonly injured)
- ACL (commonly injured)
- PCL (rarely injured)
- LCL (rarely injured)

The medial and lateral collateral ligaments lie relatively close to the skin on the inner and outer part of the knee, respectively. The medial ligament (MCL) is the most commonly injured ligament in the knee. It is injured when the upper leg is straight while the lower leg is rotated outward, as when catching the tip of a ski or when the knee is struck from the side as in a tackle (fig. 4.2). At the other extreme, the LCL, which rests on the outside of the knee, is rarely injured.

WATER ON THE KNEE

People with knee pain commonly feel that the knee is warm and swollen even if the heat is not detectable and the swelling is not visible to an outside observer. However, some patients truly have visible swelling, which is particularly true in someone who has twisted his or her knee. When the knee appears swollen, the orthopedist will want to differentiate between a knee that is simply puffy and one that is filled like a water balloon. A knee that is puffy is akin to a sponge that has absorbed water: If you put a needle in it, you will not extract fluid. This kind of swelling is common with any sprain, whether it is a knee, ankle, or finger injury. True water on the knee is a condition in which fluid fills the joint in the same way that water fills a vase. The medical term for water on the knee is *effusion.* The knee feels like a water balloon. The "water" can simply be an excessive amount of so-called joint fluid, fluid that is present in every joint. Such fluid accumulation is not harmful.

> Water on the knee in itself is not harmful.

People who suffer from arthritis are subject to this type of fluid collection, which is a reaction to the irritating by-products of arthritis and is the equivalent of an eye tearing from a speck of dust. If one removes the fluid, it often comes right back. In the case of an injury, though, the water can actually be blood. The presence of such blood suggests to the doctor that the injury may in fact be more serious than a simple sprain. Removing excess blood from the joint can also alleviate some of the pain.

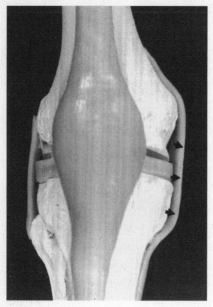

Fig. 4.1. The medial collateral ligament (MCL; black arrows). This ligament is commonly injured, but the injury rarely warrants surgery.

THE MEDIAL COLLATERAL LIGAMENT (MCL)

The MCL can be injured with one of three degrees of severity:

Grade I: The ligament is mildly stretched.
Grade II: The ligament has been considerably stretched but is still in one piece.
Grade III: The ligament has been stretched and torn into two pieces.

MCL Sprain

An MRI is not necessary to diagnose this condition!

Fig. 4.2. Injuries to the MCL.

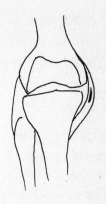

A. Grade I. Very painful, but the knee is not rendered unstable.

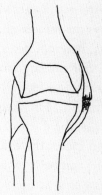

B. Grade II. With each step, the subject feels some "give" in the knee.

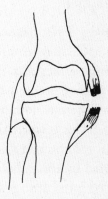

C. Grade III. Very unstable. With each step the knee opens like a hinge.

Since each of these injuries is very painful, most people readily accept the concept that they have suffered a serious injury that requires an MRI and an operation. Wrong!

Testing

By and large, an MCL injury is easily diagnosed by a physical examination and it does not require an MRI. But it does call for a physical examination, and I would not try to diagnose it on your own. Only in an athlete with a strict time schedule is it worth getting an MRI right after an injury: Indeed, there is always the remote chance that other injuries, such as a torn cartilage, may not be evident upon physical examination.

For the large majority of people, though, the most reasonable (cost-effective) course is to let the symptoms of the injury diminish. The knee is rehabilitated, and over the next two weeks, the doctor can establish whether there seems to be more than meets the eye. To the unscrupulous doctor, however, the MRI can be very useful (see below).

Treatment

Surgery is not necessary. On occasion, a severe grade III tear of the MCL may require surgical reconstruction, but this is the exception rather than the rule. Sometimes the LK-SS (see chapter 1) surgeon recommends an arthroscopic surgery "just to make sure" there is nothing else injured that might need fixing. Beware: This is where the unethical doctor will order an MRI and then recommend surgery based on the torn cartilage that is reported by the radiologist. As noted in previous chapters, a so-called torn cartilage is a common finding in normal knees and does not automatically indicate the need for surgery.

Knee Sprains and Bruises

Apply a cold pack for the first forty-eight hours, then heat.

As with any injury, your doctor will recommend the application of cold packs for the first forty-eight hours, followed by the use of heat. The cold helps to minimize swelling, most of which will have occurred within forty-eight hours. Cold can be in the form of an ice pack or a gel pack that has been placed in the freezer. Cold packs should not be applied directly to the skin. Believe it or not, you can get frostbite! Rather, place a thin towel between the cold pack and the skin. Even better: Obtain an elastic wrap (e.g., Ace), wrap it once around the knee, place the ice pack against the elastic, and finish wrapping the elastic around the cold pack. This way you don't have to hold the cold pack in place. Better yet: A surgical-supply store can probably sell you a neoprene-type sleeve equipped with pockets and gel packs. Once they are cold, just put the gel packs in the pockets and fasten the sleeve. In this situation (i.e., that of an injury), I would apply the cold pack around the clock—to the extent that it is practical for you. If the pack won't stay on while you are sleeping, don't deprive yourself of sleep just to apply an ice pack!

It is best not to use heat during the first forty-eight hours; in contrast to cold, it may increase the swelling. Once the forty-eight hours are up, though, heat is safe. It is soothing and helps you bend and straighten that painful knee. You can use the same gel packs that you had used for cold. Simply place them in hot water rather than in the freezer. Heating pads are acceptable, but don't fall asleep on them! Burns can occur. Dry heat or moist heat? It doesn't matter. Use what works best for you. There is no limit to how long you should apply the heat.

Little secret: Every now and then, even after the forty-eight hours are up, reapply the cold pack. It's a good painkiller. Alternating between heat and cold is not a problem.

Work on completely straightening the knee and bending it. You won't break anything. An injured knee wants to stay in a slightly bent position and doesn't want to be moved from that position. If you let it be, it will stiffen and tend to get stuck in that position. This stiffness may not be permanent, but it might take quite a bit of physical therapy to reverse.

How much pain should you be in? The first twenty-four to forty-eight hours are painful, and you will want a narcotic, such as codeine, oxycodone, or hydrocodone, which the doctor can prescribe. The narcotic masks the pain, and there is nothing wrong with that in this setting! Narcotics can cause drowsiness and/or constipation. It's not a bad idea to take fruit juice, even milk of magnesia, or some other laxative. This approach works best before the problem sets in!

Medications

Narcotics at first
+
anti-inflammatory medication
+
acetaminophen
(Some products combine these.)

Note that besides relieving pain at rest, pain medications allow you to perform the bending and straightening exercises described above.

In addition to narcotics, I recommend taking an anti-inflammatory medication unless there is a medical contra-indication. This type of medication is abbreviated NSAID (nonsteroidal anti-inflammatory drug). You probably think that the anti-inflammatory medication will affect the swelling. It will not. The anti-inflammatory medication cuts down the pain and swelling at the microscopic level and diminishes pain by reducing the chemical irritation that takes place after an injury. Like the army and the navy, the narcotics and the anti-inflammatory medications complement each other. In this situation, they should be used in tandem. Anti-inflammatory medications are available over the counter in a weaker form. I would ask your doctor exactly how much you should take or have him or her give you a prescription. There are medications that combine a narcotic and an anti-inflammatory drug, but as of this writing, these are brand rather than generic medications, and they tend to be considerably more expensive.

> **Anti-inflammatory medications** are not designed to control swelling. They **control pain** by blocking painful chemicals.

Medical contraindications to anti-inflammatory drugs include gastrointestinal ulcers, bleeding disorders, the taking of blood thinners, and of course, allergies or intolerance to specific anti-inflammatories.

As long as you are not suffering from side effects, you can take the NSAID medication for the few weeks that your knee can be expected to be painful. When the knee feels better, you can gradually decrease the frequency with which you take the medication.

Brand versus generic medication

I am surprised by the number of doctors who prescribe new, brand-name (i.e., expensive) anti-inflammatory medication as their first choice. Clearly they aren't paying for them! By and large, there is no difference in efficacy between a new NSAID and one whose patent has run out. Time-tested anti-inflammatory medications include naproxen, ibuprofen, sulindac, piroxicam, diclofenac, and meclofenamate—to name a few. The patents have long run out on these excellent medications, and they are no longer promoted in their original form by their parent company. They are certainly effective, and you are not likely to wake up tomorrow to find that they have been pulled off the market. For the majority of people with knee pain, one of these medications should be prescribed first.

NSAIDs can be differentiated from each other mainly by their strength and by their half-life (a measure of how long the drug stays in your body). For example, ibuprofen is short-acting and needs to be taken three or four times a day, around the clock, to be effective. Piroxicam is at the other extreme: It just needs to be taken once a day. On the other hand, ibuprofen works faster and is therefore preferable when someone is injured and requires quick relief. The prescription dose of ibuprofen is 600 milligrams three to four times a day.

> The newest anti-inflammatory medications are not stronger, just milder on the stomach.

COX-2 inhibitors. A new type of anti-inflammatory medication, it blocks one of the chemicals that causes pain without blocking the chemicals that protect the stomach. Thus, it is less likely to cause stomach ulcers and bleeding than the more traditional anti-inflammatory medications. Until their patent runs out, these NSAIDs will be rather expensive and, in my opinion, should be reserved for people who are at risk for ulcers. This includes people over fifty-five to sixty years of age and those with a history of stomach problems.

Acetaminophen (Tylenol). Once the pain of the injury has diminished, this can be a very effective (and cost-effective) medication. It *can* be taken with an NSAID. In fact, when an NSAID is allowed, I recommend adding acetaminophen. It attacks pain by way of a different chemical path and complements that of an NSAID (see my army-navy analogy on page 49). Many narcotic preparations, in fact, include acetaminophen (e.g., Tylenol #3, Percocet, Norco, Zydone), a testament to its efficacy.

Ultram. This pain reliever is in a category by itself. It is neither an NSAID nor a narcotic, and it is stronger than acetaminophen. It is more expensive than first-line medications, and in my experience, a number of people do not tolerate it. For the select patient, though, it is a good choice.

Braces. Although no bone is broken in an MCL tear, it can sure feel that way. A *brace* can make it less painful to place one's foot on the ground. The kind of braces you need for an MCL injury can be found in any surgical-supply store (a place that sells canes, crutches, and the like). The average pharmacy won't carry these items but can point you in the right direction. The braces should cost under a hundred dollars and may or may not be reimbursed by your insurance plan.

Phase 1 (first week or two). Initially, the best brace to apply is a so-called knee immobilizer, which goes from the top of the thigh down to the ankle. As the name implies, it does not allow the knee to bend. It fastens with Velcro straps and is therefore easy to put on and remove. You will want this appliance for one to two weeks. You will need it most when you walk, and you will probably also want to use it at night, as simply catching your foot on the sheets can be quite painful. It can be removed when you sit, want to bend your knee, or wash.

Knee Immobilizers

If you don't get the right length, the brace will be uncomfortable or ineffective.

Beware: Immobilizers come in different lengths, from approximately twelve to twenty-four inches. If your immobilizer is too long, it will dig into your groin and/or irritate your ankle.

If it is too short, it won't adequately support you and will not provide sufficient pain relief. Ideally, the immobilizer should start at the upper thigh and come down to two inches above your anklebone. Some immobilizers have built-in pouches for hot and cold gel packs, which are beneficial.

Certain immobilizers feature a locking-unlocking hinge. The hinge can be locked by the patient when he or she wishes support (as when walking) and be unlocked when the person wishes to bend the knee (as when sitting). Such braces will cost from two hundred to three hundred dollars and, again, will only be necessary for ten days to two weeks. Is the extra convenience worth the cost? Not for most people—at least not those paying out of pocket.

Phase 2. As the pain subsides over the two weeks following the injury, you will no longer need the knee immobilizer, but you will still benefit from some support. A hinged brace is now ideal. A somewhat short brace, it features a hinge on both sides of the knee. The hinge allows the knee to bend while protecting the knee from side-to-side forces. Such forces can be expected to remain painful for at least another month.

The Return to Sports

This is simple: You can return when you feel up to it. The knee should be pain-free and should come close to having regained its normal strength and coordination. Naturally, the more severe the injury, the longer it will take. The mildest sprains keep you out about three weeks; the more severe ones, about three months. At first, you will wear the hinged brace during sports, and gradually you will wean yourself from it. Sports involving little or no twisting will be easier to resume. Thus, running, biking, jumping rope, and swimming are easier (and safer) to engage in than football, basketball, squash, volleyball, or tennis. For tennis players, clay-type surfaces are more forgiving than concrete, since the foot is less likely to stick to the ground when the body and leg turn.

Prevention

A ligament is a very special rope, but it is nevertheless a rope. Therefore, it is difficult to condition it. On the other hand, the knee is also surrounded by strong muscles. With proper conditioning, these muscles can be strengthened and programmed to react quickly. Therefore, in certain injuries, the muscles can help control the knee and diminish the chance of an MCL tear.

The use of a hinged brace (see above) should also decrease the chance of an MCL injury and is recommended for people who have already injured this ligament. Athletes most at risk are skiers and football players. Generally, though, the use of knee braces to prevent injury is controversial. I formally recommend this only to athletes who are cautious due to a prior injury.

Skiers tend to injure their knees on the proverbial last run of the day, which has always amused me because any kind of knee injury turns a ski run into a "last run." It is true, however, that the majority of ski injuries occur late in the day. When we ran a sports clinic at the base of Hunter Mountain in New York, the late afternoon was always the busiest time. There are numerous reasons for this, including flatter, light, icier conditions and the fact that skiers are more tired at the end of the day. Muscles fatigue and become less able to quickly contract and protect ligaments such as the MCL. Therefore, Quit While You're Ahead remains a good adage for injury prevention. A conditioning program is useful for both treatment and prevention. It starts with stretching (fig. 4.3). When observed under a microscope, ligaments and tendons resemble springlike coils. Through slow and steady tension, these springs can be partially uncoiled. The operative phrase here is "slow and steady." Tension that is strong and sudden will simply result in tearing the structure, which is, of course, what happens in an injury. A stretch should be held for twenty seconds to effectively elongate those little coils.

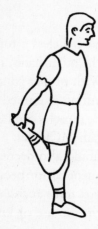

Fig. 4.3. Stretching of the quadriceps muscles.

The more these so-called soft tissues are stretched prior to athletics, the less likely they are to snap when they are suddenly stressed. The structures in the front of the knee are stretched by bringing the heel to the buttock with the hip in the extended (non-bent) position. This exercise can be carried out in the standing position. The structures in the back of the thigh (hamstrings) are stretched by touching the toes without bending the knees. This can be done standing or sitting on the ground. *Careful:* This maneuver also stretches another important rope—the sciatic nerve. This nerve runs from the spine, down the buttock, and down the back of the leg. A healthy nerve can be gently stretched in the manner described, but a sciatic nerve that is irritated for any reason will not take kindly to this type of expansion. Therefore, stretching of the hamstrings should not be carried out if pain ensues.

More sophisticated stretching involves the so-called iliotibial band, which runs along the outside of the leg (see fig. 11.6). The inside part of the leg is addressed by way of stretching the adductors, the muscles that run along the inside of the thigh. These tendons span the hip joint, not the knee joint, and therefore are of limited benefit when it comes to protecting the MCL. Nevertheless, the adductors are also subject to sudden stretching injuries when a person lunges to the side, as when reaching for a tennis ball. The adductors, therefore, deserve to be part of any stretching program.

THE ANTERIOR CRUCIATE LIGAMENT (ACL)

This has become a very fashionable ligament. Mention an ACL injury at a cocktail party and you receive grave nods of approval. Everybody recognizes it as an athlete's injury, and it puts one in the category of the elite skier, football player, and basketball player. You might even have one of those large, glitzy knee braces that come in any number of designer patterns and colors. If you're a teenager, you'll demand one.

The Historical Perspective

The pendulum often swings one way and then the other before a happy medium is reached. Until twenty years ago, the medical profession did not take ACL injuries very seriously. There were four reasons for this: (1) MRIs did not exist, nor did arthroscopies, so a number of tears were altogether missed. (2) People with a torn ACL either felt perfectly well or at most had a "trick knee," one that goes in and out when the leg is twisted in a certain way. In short, most people could (and still can) live with a torn ACL and indeed have done so since the beginning of time. (3) There didn't seem to be any long-term problems associated with this injury. (4) There were no good operations available.

We now know that a torn ACL predisposes the knee to further meniscal (cartilage) tears and can lead to arthritis. Moreover, the ACL can currently be reconstructed without resorting to lengthy incisions about the knee. This has led to a remarkable flurry of ACL surgery, some of which is unnecessary. See below.

Where Is the ACL and What Does It Do?

As noted at the beginning of this chapter, the knee is inherently unstable; it is totally dependent on ligaments and other soft tissues to stay in place.

Contrary to the MCL, which runs close to the skin, the ACL lies deep inside the knee. It courses obliquely from the outer part of the thighbone at the back of the knee down to the tablelike portion of the upper shinbone (figs. 4.4 A-C). The ACL prevents the knee from hyperextending (bending backward) and from becoming unhinged during certain twisting motions.

Fig. 4.4. The anterior cruciate ligament.

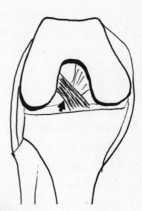

A. The normal ACL.
The PCL courses
obliquely behind it.

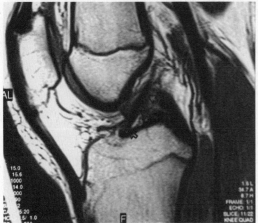

B. The normal ACL
as it appears on an
MRI.

C. A torn ACL.

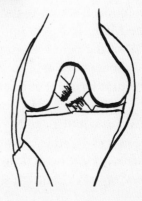

> The ACL keeps the knee from shifting during twisting motions. Its absence is more noticeable in some people than in others.

The ACL can be likened to a cable made of many strands. These strands are visible to the naked eye and can be seen to subtly twist around each other. There is some elasticity to these fibers, and therefore some give when the knee is pushed too far. Some people are loose-jointed, and by definition, their ligaments tend to have more stretch. Such people are less likely to tear their ACL, but conversely, in the event of such an injury, the other ligaments are less able to pick up the slack.

How Do You Injure an ACL?

By and large a significant injury is required to tear an ACL. You don't tear an ACL while getting up from the floor, as you might a meniscus (see chapter 3). The knee has to be forcibly twisted or hyperextended. Skiing, soccer, and football produce these typical injuries. The typical ski injury involves falling onto the back of a ski as the tip of the ski veers off to the side. Tackling in football, soccer, rugby, and related sports can lead to a tear of the MCL. It "opens up" the inside of the knee; that is, the left side of the right knee or the right side of the left knee. If a force continues to be applied to the knee and the knee keeps opening, the next ligament at risk for rupture is the ACL. (Ouch, it hurts just to think of it.) Generally speaking, it takes more force to tear an ACL than an MCL, but ACL tears without trauma have been seen in athletes who suddenly pivot as they run. The athlete with a torn ACL usually feels a pop and/or notices rapid swelling of the knee. If fluid is drained from the knee, it is usually bloody. On examination, the tibia (shinbone) can be pulled forward. This is called the "drawer" maneuver and when performed slightly differently can also be called the Lachman maneuver. The doctor may also try a "pivot" test, whereby the tibia snaps in and out of place as the knee is carefully manipulated.

Can You Prevent an ACL Injury?

By training for a particular activity you can decrease the odds of suffering an ACL injury, but you cannot eliminate the risk. High-level athletes tear this ligament with alarming frequency. No brace protects a knee from this injury, and if it existed, it would probably be too cumbersome and expensive to be prescribed on a routine basis.

Why Are Women More at Risk?

One hears surprisingly little about this on a daily basis, even though there have been numerous scientific articles and presentations about this subject. The issue of women's increased risk for major ligament injuries has even been the subject of a featured article in *Sports Illustrated*. Women have been found to be at particular risk in basketball and soccer. Other sports have been less thoroughly evaluated. Depending on the study and the setting in which women were being followed, women have been found to be anywhere from three to ten times more at risk for a tear of the ACL.

> Sport for sport *women* are at far greater risk of tearing their ACL!

Theories of the discrepancy between men and women have most recently centered on joint laxity, hormonal variations of the menstrual cycle, reaction times (how quickly muscles react to an event), and body position. (See chapter 10 for more on this.) Strength per se does not seem to be an issue. The sooner an answer is found, the sooner steps can be taken to bridge the gap. It is not clear to me to what extent women and girls who participate in these sports are aware of this phenomenon, that is, to what extent they and their parents are informed consumers. This is a particular concern in younger women, since they are the ones most likely to need surgery. It may be politically incorrect to even bring up the subject.

Not everyone needs surgery.

Factors to consider:
- age
- twisting activities
- symptoms

Do You Need Surgery?

A number of you will have zoomed right to this section. If you've had an ACL injury, it is what is uppermost in your mind. And the answer is . . . It depends. If you are an adolescent, the answer is unequivocally yes, though you might wait until you've just about stopped growing (see below). The answer is also yes if you perform jumping/twisting activities, since the ACL is a major stabilizer of the knee in those situations.

The same is also true if your knee is unstable as a result of the injury. At the other extreme, if you are over forty years old, symptom-free, and all your athletic activities are of the low impact, straight-ahead variety, such as cycling, swimming, and intermediate hiking, surgery is not necessary. Everyone in between presents a dilemma. You have to weigh the risk of surgery against perhaps being at increased risk for arthritis in the future. For if you have no symptoms from your injury, future arthritis is the only issue. As noted above, the abnormal mechanics of the knee that result from the injury can, in some people, lead to arthritis (wearing out of the articular cartilage). As of this writing, the medical profession is not able to predict who will and who will not develop arthritis as a result of an ACL tear. A concomitant tear of the meniscus (cartilage) increases the risk—especially if a large piece is torn and needs to be removed.

When this instability is added to that caused by the ACL tear, the combination appears to be too much for the knee to handle, and arthritis ensues. Another risk factor appears to be a bone bruise seen on an MRI. Such a bruise indicates that the knee took a significant hit at the time of the injury. A bruise can lead to a "hot" bone scan (formally called a nuclear technetium scan). For this test, a lightly radioactive material is injected intravenously. The technetium is mainly absorbed by bony tissue. When much of it is absorbed in one ("hot") spot, it indicates a great deal of bony activity. The hot spot reflects the body's attempt to repair the bony damage that was incurred at the time of the ACL tear. Some orthopedists feel that these bruises in and of themselves lead to an increased risk of arthritis. If that is correct, reconstructing the ACL of patients with bone bruises may not prevent arthritis! Welcome to the convoluted world of ACL tears.

On occasion, the ligament is partially torn: It appears slightly stretched, or just some of the fibers appear torn. This leads to a treatment dilemma: leave it or reconstruct it? The surgeon has to determine whether his reconstructed ligament will be better than your imperfect ACL. I tend to err on leaving the patient's own ligament unless the patient's symptoms can be explained only by the partial tear.

If you fall into the large group of patients for whom the operation may or may not be indicated, only *you* can make the decision as to whether to have surgery or not. There is no right answer, only what is right for you. Whichever road you choose, you should embark upon it with confidence. You will be happier with the results.

When Should Surgery Be Performed?

Is it better to operate on the knee when it has just been seriously traumatized, or is it better to wait for the knee to recover somewhat before assaulting it again? You can argue this all day. Needless to say, orthopedists in ski resorts see things somewhat differently from their colleagues in the cities. As a city orthopedist, I would rather let the athlete adjust to the physical and emotional aspect of the trauma, collect his or her wits, search the Internet, make the appropriate work/school arrangements, rehab the knee to restore reasonable strength and motion, and then peacefully and carefully reconstruct the ligament. In cities, as in mountains resorts, a number of orthopedists use the shoe-salesman approach described in the previous chapter: Sign up the patient for surgery right away or risk losing the patient. After all, in a few weeks the patient may feel well and refuse surgery altogether. In that case, the surgeon no longer gets the credit for the patient's recovery.

ACL Injuries in Adolescents

This is not as controversial as it used to be. Children whose ACL has been torn do not do well. The problem is that surgery of a torn ACL involves making holes in the bones about the knee, which happens to be where the major growth plates are. Surgery performed through these growth plates might affect the growth of the bone. This is particularly true in children with much growth left and is of lesser importance in those whose growth is nearly complete. In the setting of the child with wide-open growth plates, soft-tissue grafts, such as the "hamstring" graft, may be less likely to harm the growth plates than the patellar-tendon graft, which includes a piece of bone at both ends (see below).

Types of Graft:

- patellar tendon
- gracilis/semitendinosis ("hamstring")
- quadriceps tendon
- allograft
- synthetic

Types of Surgery

When something is torn, the natural reaction is to sew it back together. Therefore, the earliest operations for a torn ACL involved sewing the torn ends, which did not work. Perhaps the techniques were inadequate, or perhaps a stretched and torn cablelike structure is simply not amenable to sewing. In any case, the current party line is that an ACL cannot be fixed. If instead of being torn the ligament has been pulled off at its origin on the thighbone, some will argue that it can be reattached to its origin, much as an anchor can be pushed back into the sand after it has been pulled out. But it is not accepted practice, which is not to say that it is wrong.

In all likelihood, the surgeon will offer you a reconstruction whereby another structure will be used to replace the torn ligament. This structure can be from your own body (an *autograft*), it can come from a bone bank—an elegant way of saying that it comes from a cadaver (an *allograft*)—or it can be *synthetic*. Synthetics are naturally the most appealing, but those that have been tried in the United States have not worked.

Allografts have the obvious advantage over autografts, since they leave your own body intact. You're not sacrificing any part of your body. But cadaveric allografts are expensive, and more significantly, there is always the small chance that some disease will be transmitted. With your luck, the cadaver will have had some hidden, horrible disease, right? Because of this slight risk, such grafts are heavily radiated to the point where cynics have likened them to a piece of a bacon. That's not really fair, but the point is that allografts are an acceptable but not ideal solution. They tend to be used when multiple grafts are needed or when the patient is going for a second operation and an autograft has already been used in the first procedure.

All autografts sacrifice healthy, useful tissue to create a new ligament, robbing Peter to pay Paul, so to speak. In the future, we can expect to either grow a new ligament or find an acceptable synthetic ligament. In the meantime, there are three sources of autografts: the patellar tendon, the hamstring tendon, and the quadriceps tendon, in order of current popularity. The patellar-tendon graft includes the middle third of the tendon connecting your kneecap (patella) to your tibial tuberosity (the knob at the top of your shinbone) as well as a piece of bone at each end of the tendon. One piece of bone comes off the kneecap; the other, off the tuberosity (see figs. 4.5 A & B). You would think that this would leave the rest of the patellar tendon

Fig. 4.5. The ACL reconstruction with the patellar tendon.

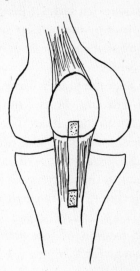

A. Graft taken from the patellar tendon at the front of the knee.

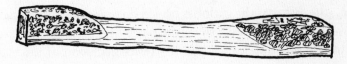

B. "Bone-patellar tendon-bone" graft.

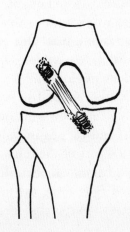

C. Fixation of the graft with screws or equivalent "hardware." Note that there are many ways of fixing a graft. They all require the use of a metallic or plasticlike device.

quite weakened and prone to rupture, but with cautious rehabilitation, that has not been the case. This is fortunate because
a rupture of the patellar tendon is an orthopedic disaster re-
quiring at the very least one major operation and a long period
of recovery.

Once the graft is harvested, it has to be placed inside the
knee. For this, holes ("tunnels") are created, and the graft is
passed into those holes. The graft has to be locked to one of the
tunnels, made taut, and finally, fixed to the other tunnel (fig.
4.5 C). The advantage of having a piece of bone at either end of
the graft is that a screw can be placed in the tunnels, thus wedg-
ing the bone from the graft to the walls of the tendon. Recently,
so-called soft tissue screws have become available. These permit
screw fixation of soft grafts, such as patellar or quadriceps-
tendon grafts. Within a few months, the graft is forever secured.
Unfortunately, as Jerry Rice of the San Francisco 49ers will tell
you, the fact that the graft has healed does not mean that the recovery is over. The host site—the place that the graft was taken
from—needs time to recover. If stressed too soon or too vigor-
ously, the kneecap may fracture, or the remaining tendon may
rupture. The rope that was just placed in the knee also needs
time to start looking and acting like an ACL. Opinions are divided as to how long this takes. Some say two years, but nobody
wants to wait that long. The party line is one year. One year,
therefore, before resuming contact sports. The very long-term
effects of harvesting a graft of any kind are not known.

You have three hamstring muscles: the biceps (the same
name as the muscle in your arm), which runs down the outer
part of your thigh, the semitendinosus, and the semimembra-
nosus, both of which run along the back part of the thigh. In
the *hamstring graft*, the semitendinosus is harvested, often along
with another tendon, the gracilis, which runs along the inner
thigh (fig. 4.6). These tendons are there for a purpose, so for the

surgeon it is emotionally painful to sacrifice them. Yet athletes appear to function well even after the harvesting of these tendons. There is less donor-site morbidity, as we say in medical lingo, than with the patellar tendon. Nothing bad is going to happen to the site from which the graft was taken if the athlete makes a hasty return to sports. As with all grafts, there are umpteen ways of fixing a hamstring graft to the bone, but they

Fig. 4.6. The ACL reconstruction with "hamstrings"

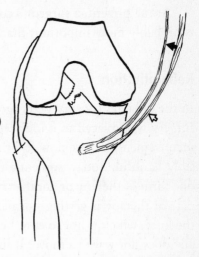

A. Semitendinosus (hamstring) tendon and gracilis tendon.

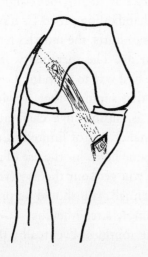

B. Fixation of the "hamstring" graft. There is a small metallic button on the femur (thighbone) and a metallic staple on the tibia (shinbone). This is just one of many ways of fixing the graft.

all involve hardware—a screw, a staple, etc. Some of this hardware can be absorbable. Instead of being metallic, it is made of a dissolvable material. These products are still evolving.

The quadriceps tendon joins the quadriceps muscles at the front of your thigh to the kneecap. The *quadriceps-tendon graft* has some of the advantages and disadvantages of the other two grafts and is equally acceptable.

At the present, a surgeon's comfort level with a certain graft is probably more important than the graft itself.

Rehabilitation

In the old days (twenty years ago), people undergoing ligament surgery were placed in a long leg cast. Not only was it terribly inconvenient, but we now feel that it was unnecessary and possibly harmful. Today, someone undergoing ACL surgery starts one form of therapy or another right away. The most important part of therapy is getting normal bending and straightening of the knee, which is not so easy, because the operated knee generally does not want to move. It likes to stay slightly bent and to be left alone. For some people, the rehabilitation process is more difficult than for others. When the knee hurts, the muscles tend to atrophy, and the tendons tighten up. The therapist works with you to reverse that process. The best way to train for a certain activity is to perform exercises that simulate that activity. Therefore, isokinetic exercises, that is, sitting in a chair and straightening your leg against a resistance, are of limited value after the initial recovery phase. The same holds for the use of an exercise bicycle. Regardless of where you get your therapy (yes, some form of physical therapy is essential), you should be progressing from motion exercises to simple strengthening movements to more sophisticated exercise routines. Eventually, the therapist elaborates a program for you that you can carry out at home or at the gym.

Return to Sports

Some patients are satisfied with simply having a stable knee during everyday activities, but most patients with ACL tears want to go back to sports. Activities that put the reconstructed ligament at risk are the same ones that led to the ACL tear in the first place: uncontrolled jumping and twisting. They are therefore the last to be permitted. On the other hand, simple running, jumping in place with both feet, and even side-to-side jumping are allowed early on. Swimming is also admissible in the early going.

Can the New, Surgically Reconstructed ACL Rupture, Too?

You bet. A paradox of sports medicine is that we operate on knees so that athletes can go back to the sports they love, yet those very activities can lead to a rupture of the new ACL. Since the new ACL is a relatively crude version of the original, it is easier to tear than the original. And as with all operations, the surgery the second time around is far more complex than the first one. As bitter a pill as it is to swallow, the person who doesn't earn a living from sports might consider toning down his or her activities after an ACL reconstruction.

THE POSTERIOR CRUCIATE AND LATERAL (FIBULAR) COLLATERAL LIGAMENTS

Injuries to these ligaments are far less common but potentially far more serious. The posterior cruciate ligament lies in the center of the knee, where it crosses behind its anterior counterpart, the ACL. It shares some functions with the ACL to the extent that it helps provide smooth, controlled motion of the knee. It does so, however, in a manner just opposite the ACL, which is understandable considering that one goes from top right to bottom left, so to speak, and the other goes from top left to bottom right (see fig. 4.4). The PCL prevents the thighbone from sliding forward when one goes down steps, and as with the ACL, it prevents abnormal twisting.

The lateral collateral ligament (LCL), also called fibular collateral ligament, is the equivalent of the MCL: It lies relatively close to the skin along the outer aspect of the knee. In a manner similar to the MCL, its origin is on the femur, but instead of inserting on the upper tibia, as does the MCL, it inserts on top of the fibula, the skinny bone on the outer aspect of the leg.

Whereas the MCL is the most commonly injured ligament, the LCL is arguably the least commonly injured. This is fortunate, because when the LCL is torn, the PCL is commonly torn, too (and vice versa), and this combination always mandates surgery. It will not heal on its own, and left untreated, it will lead to a very unstable knee.

Isolated PCL tears are quite rare, and the necessity to address this problem surgically is more controversial. Many patients with an isolated PCL tear do not even realize that they have a torn ligament. An isolated PCL tear can occur when the tibia is forcibly pushed backward. Landing with your shin on a log, for example, will push the shin bone backward relative to the knee. Rarely, hitting the leg against the dashboard will push the leg back in such a way as to tear the PCL. (This is not an excuse for getting an MRI of everyone who hits his or her knee on a dashboard!) An isolated PCL tear may be asymptomatic and therefore does not automatically mandate surgery. But in young, athletic people, a torn PCL probably leads to subtle abnormal motions and is probably best reconstructed. This is the injury sustained by the notable quarterback Randall Cunningham before his resounding comeback with the Minnesota Vikings. Note that, once again, a PCL cannot be repaired, that is, stitched back together. As with the ACL, it needs to be reconstructed with another structure. Because the PCL tends to be torn along with other structures (ACL and/or LCL), chances are that an allograft (see above paragraph on ACL surgery) will be used for part of the reconstruction.

Isolated LCL injuries are distinctly unusual and, most of the time, require surgery.

Fortunately, we live in an era in which these injuries can be detected and a surgical solution, albeit imperfect, can be offered.

Chapter 5

"Urgent" Arthritis Surgery

THERE IS NO URGENT ARTHRITIS SURGERY. BUT THAT IS NOT the sense I get from certain patients. They have seen an orthopedist who has told them that the X rays look bad and that they should have surgery—soon.

WHAT IS ARTHRITIS?

A shiny white material lines the end of each bone. Check it out the next time you eat chicken. This material is called cartilage. Specifically, it is articular cartilage. The term *articular* differentiates it from meniscal cartilage, the rubbery shock absorber described in chapter 3. The term *torn cartilage* refers to meniscal cartilage and has *nothing to do with arthritis*.

Arthritis has a specific definition: *the wearing of articular cartilage down to the bone* (figs. 5.1 A & B). There have been

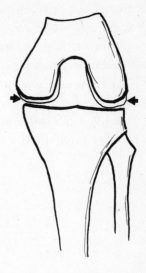

Fig. 5.1A. The ends of the bones are covered with a smooth, glistening white material that is six times more slippery than ice. This is called *articular cartilage* (solid arrows).

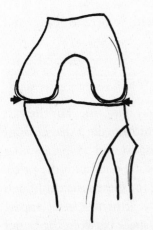

Fig. 5.1B. A joint is said to be arthritic when the cartilage has completely worn down over any part of the joint. When this occurs, the bones come together. This is good for people but not for bones.

many controversies in the history of arthritis, but the above definition is not one of them.[1]

Arthritis can have multiple causes. These include a genetically caused deterioration of the cartilage; a mechanical overload

1. There are variations on the word *arthritis. Arthrosis* is also used, and purists like to argue the relative merits of both terms.

of the cartilage, as when people are very bowlegged or knock-kneed; trauma—a severe whack to the cartilage or a fracture through the cartilage; an infection; or a rheumatological condition. A rheumatological condition is one in which the lining of the joint secretes a product that slowly degrades the articular cartilage (see also chapter 6).

Arthritis can involve just one small part of the knee, or it can be more generalized.

THE ROLE OF X RAYS

There are four major misconceptions with respect to X rays and arthritis.

Misconception 1

You really need an MRI, not an X ray. Not true. For the vast majority of people, an X ray is sufficient to make a diagnosis of arthritis (figs. 5.2 A & B). It is upsetting to find people coming to me with an MRI when an X ray, costing one-tenth the price, would have sufficed. We are all paying for these tests! Although cartilage does not show up on an X ray, arthritis can be apparent on an X ray in different ways: The space between the bones becomes narrower, a sign that the cartilage is wearing thin. In extreme cases, the bones are seen to touch each other. This indicates that the cartilage is completely worn out. Another radiographic sign of arthritis is the presence of bone spurs, called osteophytes. These look like little rose thorns, and they tell the doctor, "Look over here. There's worn cartilage in the neighborhood."

Four X-ray and MRI Misconceptions

1. X rays aren't good enough—you need an MRI.
2. Arthritis is always detected by an MRI.
3. Arthritis on an X ray means a person is suffering.
4. Arthritis on an X ray means a person needs surgery.

Misconception 2

Any arthritis can be seen on an MRI. Not true. If the arthritis is localized in one or more small areas, it can escape detection. This is a frequent source of frustration and anger in patients who undergo an outpatient knee procedure and are told after the surgery that they have arthritis. As far as they are concerned, the arthritis should have been detected preoperatively. The truth is that the possible existence of arthritis should indeed have been discussed preoperatively, but arthritis may not have been detectable on an MRI.

Misconception 3

If the arthritis looks bad on an X ray, the person must be suffering quite a bit. Again, not true. My favorite story is that of a ninety-plus-year-old man who came in to talk about his knees. The X rays he put on my desk revealed some of the worst arthritis I have ever seen. There was absolutely no space between the bones, and there were huge bone spurs. I braced myself for a discussion of knee replacement surgery in nonagenarians. Then the gentleman put forth his complaint: He liked to carry his own golf bag when playing golf and was now finding that after eighteen holes his knees were "sore." That was it. Sore. Here was a man walking and playing eighteen holes of golf on one of the most horrible knees I'd ever seen. Meanwhile, some people with a fraction of his arthritis can barely walk! Why arthritis causes more pain in some people than in others remains one of the mysteries of the condition.

Misconception 4

If the arthritis looks bad on an X ray, surgery is indicated. Once again, not true. The following is a common ploy: The LK-SS surgeon shows the patient that "bad" arthritis on the X ray and quickly gets the sucker, er, patient, to agree to surgery "before it's too late," so he says. This is very unscrupulous. As we have just noted, there is no correlation between how bad X rays look and how a person might feel. Moreover, surgery should not be considered unless all reasonable nonoperative alternatives have failed. Finally, the arthritis pain may subside on its own (see below).

The Proper X-Rays

Standard X rays performed by an emergency room or by a health professional without a particular interest in knees will include a *front and side view* of your knee. For both views you lie on the X-ray table. If you have severe arthritis, these two simple views will suffice. The arthritis will be apparent, and the diagnosis will be made. For any condition other than advanced arthritis, however, these two views are likely to be inadequate.

If your knee hurts and you are over forty years old, there is a chance that you might have early arthritis involving only a small portion of your knee. In this case, at the very least, you should be standing for the frontal X ray. This increases the odds that the narrowing of your joint will be apparent.

If there is any chance that your kneecap might be contribut-

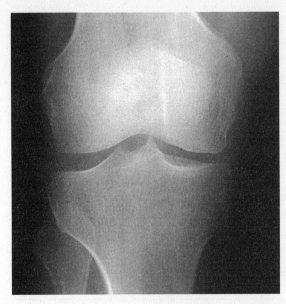

Fig. 5.2A.
A plain X ray
reveals the *joint
space narrowing.*
This is the medical
term for "bones
coming together
and rubbing." In
some people, this
is very painful.
A. A normal
X ray. Note the
space between the
bones.

Fig. 5.2B. An abnormal
X ray. Note the bones
touching on one side of
the knee. The MRI report
on this patient read first
and foremost "tear of the
medial meniscus." Yet
another misleading MRI.

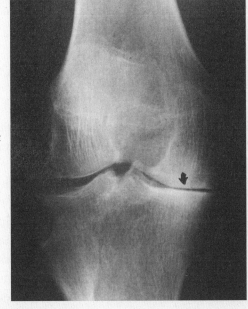

ing to your pain, which is true a significant percentage of the time, you should be getting an X ray that goes by a number of names, including "sunrise" view and Merchant view, named after Alan Merchant, M.D., from California. This view, admittedly, takes extra time, added knowledge on the part of the person taking the X ray, and some inexpensive supplementary equipment. For this view, the patient lies on his or her back, legs bent over the end of the X-ray table, resting on a special device. This device keeps the knees bent at a specified angle, usually in the 30–45-degree range. With these X rays, the doctor can determine if the kneecap is well seated in its groove (see chapter 6). The doctor can also detect arthritis that might be present under the kneecap. In some patients, arthritis is only present under the kneecap, and without this view *the arthritis will be completely missed!*

> Unless a so-called skyline or Merchant X ray is obtained, your arthritis might be completely missed!

There are other sophisticated views that can be obtained, and these are discussed in chapter 7.

Here is the point: If you are sent for two X rays of the knee—both taken lying down—and are then sent off for an MRI, chances are you are dealing with an LK-SS. Someone is wasting your time and money.

There are exceptions. If you are under the age of forty and it is very clear that the problem lies with the meniscus or one of the cruciate ligaments—neither of which show up on an X ray—it is reasonable to skip the X rays altogether and to go right for the MRI. Your insurance may force the doctor to obtain an X ray first, a foolish policy in my opinion, and in this case, it is reasonable to obtain the two simplest views.

Are MRIs a Waste of Time?

No. As noted elsewhere in this book, there are multiple sources of knee pain, some of which are best detected by an MRI. But in someone likely to have arthritis the answer is yes. If you are in your late sixties or older and you have had recurrent nagging knee pain, the chances are overwhelming that you have arthritis even if you feel otherwise quite youthful. The above-mentioned X rays will usually prove this. Even when these X rays cannot demonstrate the arthritis, it is still the most likely diagnosis in this age group. The MRI may indeed confirm the arthritis, but you need to ask yourself, is this MRI necessary, and is it worth the cost? The knowledgeable doctor will have already given you the diagnosis.

Can an MRI Be Misleading?

You bet. Not only is an MRI not necessary in the context of arthritis; it can be terribly misleading. Anyone with arthritis is likely to have a reading of a torn meniscus on their MRI. In fact, to the radiologist, the torn meniscus may be more obvious than the arthritis, and the focus of the report may be on this alleged tear (fig. 5.3). This error in focus is a major concern because, as we saw in chapter 2, the tear may or may not be real. Even if it is, the arthritis is by far the bigger problem. Imagine a house on fire and burning down. Does the firefighter care whether there is a leaky faucet in the second-floor bathroom? Does he care whether the curtains in the living room are faded and may need to be replaced? Of course not! The burning house takes precedence over everything else! Likewise, in a patient with chronic arthritis symptoms, just about any other condition detected by the MRI is likely to be trivial. In summary, the MRI in this setting muddies the waters.

> MRIs can be very misleading.

Can Pain Come and Go?

Not only can pain come and go; it *typically* comes and goes. The patient visiting the doctor with an arthritic flare-up will agree to just about anything, and the LK-SS doctor will take advantage of that by proposing surgery. On the other hand, doctors who prescribe remedies that allegedly require three months of continued use before they can be effective are taking advantage of the fact that, in that period of time, most arthritic flare-ups will have subsided on their own.

OSTEOARTHRITIS VERSUS OSTEOPOROSIS

The two words are similar, and it stands to reason that they would describe similar conditions. Sorry, there is no connection between the two. Osteoarthritis is the genetically or mechanically induced wearing out of the thin layer of cartilage at the end of a bone. Osteoporosis is a condition of bone, not cartilage, in which the bone becomes thin and fragile. Normal bone is to osteoporotic bone what dense fog is to light fog. Same stuff, less of it.

One can have osteoarthritis with or without osteoporosis and vice versa.

THE NONOPERATIVE
TREATMENT OF ARTHRITIS

Rest

This may seem obvious, but people sometimes want to work through the pain. An arthritic flare-up demands rest. Gentle exercises can be resumed once the acute pain has abated.

Heat and Cold Treatment

Although they are opposites, both heat and cold can be soothing. People generally like to be given specific formulas (e.g., "Do this for ten minutes, then do that for fifteen minutes"), but when it comes to heat and cold there is no right or wrong. It's a question of what works best for each individual person. I generally recommend ten minutes of one followed by ten minutes of the other. "Should the heat be moist or dry?" is a frequently asked question. Personally, I have not noted a difference, although individual patients have indicated a preference for one or the other. Some people, for example, feel particularly well in a warm bath. Beware of overdoing it! I've seen people *burn* themselves with a heating pad. Taking a sedative, imbibing an alcoholic beverage, and falling asleep with an electric heating pad around your knee is not a good idea. When it comes to cold, the key is not to place ice directly on the skin. Believe it or not, you can get *frostbite!* Place a towel or wrap an elastic bandage between the ice and your skin. There are some commercially available neoprene wraps that can house a gel pack. This pack can be cooled or heated. In fact, two gel packs can be used, so that while one is being used, the other can be either cooled or heated.

Medications. Part I: Oral Medications (pills)

These fall into many categories: *Analgesics* simply mask the pain. There is nothing wrong with that as long as you don't go out and abuse your arthritic joint while you're feeling better. These include acetaminophen (Tylenol) and tramadol (Ultram). Acetaminophen is an over-the-counter medication and is relatively safe. Nevertheless, it can have serious side effects that you don't even feel (e.g., liver damage), and you should inform your doctor if you find yourself taking this medication on a regular basis. (I feel that this is true for any medication or nutritional supplement.)

Anti-inflammatories outside the steroid category are abbreviated *NSAID* for "nonsteroidal anti-inflammatory drugs." These calm the pain by chemically relieving the irritation associated with arthritis. Aspirin is the granddaddy of all NSAIDs. In ancient Greece, women in labor were advised to chew on the leaves of the willow tree, as the salicin in the leaves would alleviate their pain. A salicin derivative has become the aspirin we know today. It is common wisdom that had it been discovered just in the last few decades, it would never have been approved as an over-the-counter drug. It has multiple effects, it can interact with other medications, and it can adversely affect important biological functions for many weeks. For example, aspirin compromises platelets that help the blood to clot. This is very useful when aspirin is used as a blood thinner, but it is a major problem when blood thinning is contraindicated. You should definitely let your doctor know that you are taking aspirin when he or she prescribes any other medication.

Since the introduction of aspirin, dozens of NSAIDs have appeared on, and disappeared from, the market. Each one naturally claims to be more powerful and have fewer side effects than the existing ones. These side effects include stomach ulcers, which can hurt and cause serious bleeding and more insidious damage to various organ systems, such as the kidneys. The possibility has even been raised that NSAIDs can harm articular cartilage—the very root of the arthritis problem. I have not personally noted clinical evidence of this, but it is a point worth keeping in mind. The newest class of NSAIDs is the so-called COX-2 inhibitor (Celebrex [celecoxib], Vioxx [rofecoxib], and in standard doses Mobic [meloxicam]), which is even less likely to cause ulcers than the recent NSAIDs already being touted as being mild on the stomach. Note that the COX-2 NSAIDs are not better pain relievers than the other NSAIDs. So if your current NSAID works and you are not at risk for ulcers (speak to your doctor about this), I would not switch. Not to mention that Celebrex and Vioxx are quite expensive.

The following is another common misconception: NSAIDs will reduce swelling. If the knee is swollen due to the irritation of arthritis, then yes, maybe. But if the swelling is the result of an injury, no! You might take ibuprofen, for instance, for the pain of a sprained ankle, but don't expect it to control that goose egg on the outside of your foot! NSAIDs control the pain of irritation but do not remove any water that has accumulated. The swelling from an injury will only resolve with rest, elevation, cold, compression, tincture of time [*sic*], powder of patience, and extract of expectation.

Keep in mind that patents run out after a few years. If you wonder why you don't hear of a great medication after a while, it's either because serious side effects have been discovered and the drug has been pulled off the market or, more likely, the patent has run out, and advertising is no longer cost-effective. One medication that I have found to be effective is naproxen. It is convenient (twice-a-day dosage) and has been around a very long time. In its generic form it is relatively inexpensive, and you are not likely to wake up to the news that it has been pulled from the market. Remarkably, certain HMOs and insurance companies will not cover naproxen. They will, however, cover brand-only, expensive NSAIDs. Go figure.

One point that is remarkably unappreciated is that you can combine an NSAID with an analgesic. For example, you can take naproxen with breakfast and dinner and in between add acetaminophen. (Check with your doctor for the exact dosage.)

Should you be asking for the very latest NSAID? By now, you know where I'm going with this. The obvious answer is the wrong one. Every new car model is better than the last one, but the same isn't true for medications or medical devices. True, our government demands stringent tests, but there are still surprises. Remember Duract? Of course not. It came out briefly in the late 1990s and was history before you could say "complication." People got touchy about a few deaths here and there, and in the twitch of a liver enzyme, it was gone. Mind you, there may have been a little overreaction on the part of public. It really wasn't clear that the deaths were related to the medication, but the point remains that there can be surprises with new medications.

Then there are the new medications that aren't new at all. Take the case of the pain reliever Vicoprofen. Vicoprofen consists of two separate medications put together: hydrocodone and ibuprofen. Hydrocodone is a strong, time-honored narcotic, and ibuprofen is a classic NSAID available as Motrin, Advil, Nuprin, or, well, ibuprofen. These two medications are relatively cheap as generics. *Now, here's the trick, so pay attention.* Although hydrocodone and ibuprofen are inexpensive on their own, one enterprising manufacturer has combined the two medications to create the more expensive Vicoprofen! You'd have thought, *Nah, that'll never work.* Who would pay a lot of money for a pill that consists of two inexpensive medications? Well, wrong again. This has been a popular medication. Did the doctors not recognize the ingredients? Did the drug company take unfair advantage of the confusion? Maybe for some people the convenience of swallowing one larger pill rather than two smaller ones is really worth the extra expense. You be the judge.

And by the way, Vicoprofen isn't alone. Many prescriptions and over-the-counter medications are pricey combinations of inexpensive products. Read the label and check with your pharmacist.

Steroids are a large class of medications. Steroids used for the pain of arthritis are different from anabolic steroids taken by some athletes. Cortisone was one of the original steroids, and the word cortisone is still used colloquially to denote any type of steroid. Steroids are strong anti-inflammatory medications, but they are associated with a long list of potential side effects. These include stomach ulcers, fluid retention, the raising of blood sugar, bone necrosis ("bone strokes"; see chapter 6), osteoporosis, to name but a few. Not everyone suffers from these side effects. The likelihood of developing one or more side effects depends on the dose of the medication and on the length of time the medication is taken. Despite their potential side effects, steroids are sometimes the only medications that will be effective, and doctors do still prescribe them. Interestingly, though the word cortisone is commonly used, I don't believe that it is still in clinical practice—at least not in the United States. Indeed, although cortisone conjures up nasty things in people's minds, it is actually relatively weak. Prednisone, on the other hand, is much stronger and is a commonly prescribed steroid.

An arthritic flare-up can be excruciating, and on a short-term basis it is reasonable to take a *narcotic.* In the long run, it is not advisable to use narcotics, for the reasons most of us know: They are addictive, and they become less effective with time. One is said to become tolerant of them. If you take narcotics, keep in mind that they can be constipating and can make you drowsy. *The most common narcotics are combined with acet-aminophen or aspirin.* Check the label. If your narcotic already contains acetaminophen, it is not a good idea to take even more acetaminophen. The same goes for aspirin.

Consider this little-known fact: Pain medications work best when the knee just starts to hurt. Sometimes it doesn't pay to be a hero. When you feel the pain coming on, take something for it.

Medications. Part II: Injections

As unappealing as they are to most people, knee injections still have a role. They usually consist of a combination of a numbing agent (e.g., Novocain) and a steroid. You'll be interested to know that not all steroids are equivalent. Some are more expensive than others, and in my opinion, this is an example of getting what you pay for: The more expensive ones are stronger, last longer, and don't leave a dandrufflike residue in the knee.

There are downsides to steroid injections: Not only are they not curative; they make the tissues less healthy and more prone to infection. There is therefore a limit to how many injections one can prescribe. I limit knee-joint injections to three per year. Note that injections affect the site that has been injected and have limited impact on other sites. If you've had three shoulder injections, you can still receive a knee injection.

There exists a class of injections not related to steroids. Introduced in 1998, these are injections of a gooey material similar to the hyaluronic acid that your own knee makes. Depending on the specific brand, the patient needs to come for a series of three or five weekly shots. Injecting these products into the knee is akin to adding oil to a machine. Moreover, the manufacturers have found that cartilage growth can be stimulated by these injections. It is not clear to what extent this is a clinically significant finding, in other words, to what extent people will benefit from this feature. In my experience, these injections work best in patients whose arthritis is not terribly advanced, but I have seen exceptions in both directions. These injections are pricey, and not all insurances cover them.[2]

Nutritional Supplements

The above-mentioned pills and injections do not cure arthritis; they simply quiet the pain. It would be very appealing to prescribe a medication that actually leads to the regeneration of worn-out cartilage. The manufacturers of two products—glucosamine and chondroitin sulfate—have made such a claim, and there is a school of thought that the two products should be taken together. Even the most fervent proponents recognize that the pain relief does not start until the products have been used regularly for at least one month. (Some say three months.) Since both products exist in the body, though not necessarily in that exact form, they cannot be called drugs. They are classified as nutritional supplements. The *good news* is that they are not under the control of the FDA and scientific validation is not required. They can be promoted and sold without having to wait the many years it takes for the FDA to determine that something is safe and effective. The *bad news* is that they are not under the control of the FDA and scientific validation is not required. They can be promoted and sold without having to wait the many years it takes for the FDA to determine that something is safe and effective! If the products are found to be inef-

2. Some insurance companies are devious. They claim to cover the products, but only on condition that the patient not be a candidate for a knee replacement. Yet every patient with knee arthritis is a candidate for a knee replacement! If the potential need for a replacement is in any way stated in the patient's record, coverage is denied!

fective, many people will have wasted an awful lot of money. Fortunately, so far it appears that the products are safe. I do not know of side effects of these compounds. Anecdotally, a number of my patients swear by the product. Therefore, if money is not an issue (the supplements can be expensive), I don't discourage my patients from trying them. But one has to keep in mind the fact that arthritic flare-ups subside on their own (see above) and that there can be placebo effects.

A *placebo* (from the Latin "I shall please") is a treatment that the doctor recognizes as having no medicinal value (see chapter 9). Yet if the patient believes enough in the treatment, this may be enough to ensure success. "Mind over matter." Although I am discussing this in the context of nutritional supplements, for which there has been little scientific validation, the placebo effect can be manifest with any treatment, even surgery!

Diet

Rattlesnake meat, vinegar, honey, and white meat have all been touted as arthritis remedies, whereas tomatoes, eggplant, potatoes, sweets, and dairy products get thumbs down. That is, if you believe in all this. I don't.

It would be all too easy if a rattlesnake-and-honey sandwich did the trick. Don't get me wrong. Many of our scientific remedies come from natural products. If aspirin can come from the willow tree, then perhaps there is something medicinal about honey. But if this were the case, it would no longer be a secret, and right now, if honey or vinegar is effective against arthritis, it's certainly a secret to me. "Sweetie, just a little extra vinegar on my salad and I'll join you on the tennis court!" I simply do not hear that very often.

Physical Therapy (PT)

Physical therapy is a broad field, including exercises and so-called modalities designed to promote motion and decrease pain. The exercises themselves can be divided into the stretching and the strengthening types. When physical therapy is suggested to patients with arthritis, they occasionally have the mistaken impression that they are being sent for a strengthening program, complete with pushing, pulling, huffing, and puffing. This is not appealing. However, PT in the setting of knee arthritis is more of the *stretching-and-modality* variety.

An arthritic knee tends to get stiff. This is the body's natural response to arthritis. Moving an arthritic joint is what hurts. If the knee could be rendered completely stiff to the point where it didn't move at all, there would be no pain. There are problems with the body's attempt to freeze the joint: (1) The joint is never completely stiff, and so the pain persists. (2) A stiff joint doesn't work very well. (3) The stiffness is, to some extent, imparted by the chronic tensing of muscles, and this itself can contribute to the person's pain. A portion of PT, therefore, involves restoring reasonable motion to the knee.

In addition to applying heat and cold, which patients can do on their own at home, PT can involve modalities such as ultrasound and, in more sophisticated settings, iontophoresis or phonophoresis. This is a process by which drugs are applied to the skin and electrochemically led to diffuse through the skin. In my experience, these modalities tend to work better on knee problems that are relatively superficial (e.g., tendinitis) than on arthritis, which lives down deep inside the joint. Nevertheless, it can be worth trying.

Massage. The tendons and muscles about the arthritic knee tend to be stiff and sore. Massage aids in the stretching of these structures and thereby soothes the knee. It also soothes the soul and is not an insignificant factor in the overall treatment of the patient whose pain has rendered him or her tense and irritable.

Taping. If the arthritis is confined to the kneecap and if the kneecap is poorly aligned (see X-ray section above), special taping techniques can be used to pull the kneecap toward its normal position (see chapter 6). This can take just enough pressure off the kneecap to afford some pain relief.

Exercise

Patients with knee arthritis tend not to exercise. Exercise hurts. There is also the fear that exercise will aggravate the arthritis. Nevertheless, not only is exercise allowed in this setting, it is to be encouraged—not just for the sake of the knee but for the accepted cardiovascular benefits of aerobic exercise.

> Yes, people with arthritis should exercise.

We are not talking about just any exercise. Jumping and twisting activities will tend to increase the pain. At the other extreme, *water exercises* are wonderful. The body is buoyant, and therefore, by definition, less weight is placed across the knee. Running, which on land could be painful, may suddenly be quite tolerable. It can be carried out in the shallow end of a pool or, with special flotation belts, in the deep end. Likewise, kicking and jumping exercises are more readily prescribed in water. These strengthen the muscles (which makes the knee feel more secure), stretch the structures about the knee, contribute to cardiovascular fitness, and provide a sense of well-being. The water temperature should be comfortable; if not initially, at least within a few moments of exercising. If the water is too cold, the muscles will become even more tense and painful.

For land exercises, cushioned shoes should be worn. Use of a *treadmill* is reasonable, since the surface is relatively soft. The use of an *exercise bicycle* can address stiffness if the seat is high enough, but by and large it is a neutral exercise: It won't help, and it won't hurt. Running is controversial. At one point, it was felt to cause arthritis, but recent studies suggest that in a perfectly normal knee, running does not promote arthritis. In a knee that is already arthritic, it may be a different story. I would tend to discourage running in someone who is quite bowlegged or knock-kneed.

Shoe Wear

In a painfully arthritic knee, any jarring step hurts. Classic leather-soled shoes with hard rubber heels don't help the situation. Wearing shoes with softer heels, such as running shoes, or inserting a cushioned insole can help. If you use an insole, make sure it is thick enough. Some foam insoles collapse like tissue paper and provide minimal cushioning. Silicone (not silicon) inserts are more durable and provide more cushioning.

Canes, Sticks, and the Like

Getting a patient to use a cane is a measure of how good a sales-man the doctor is. Other than orthopedic shoes, no other treatment option has such a stigma attached to it. Whereas knee-replacement surgery is high-tech, a cane just makes you look old—or so people feel. Naturally, men take to canes better than women. There are some very elegant canes, and men with canes can still conjure up a certain aura. A hiking stick may be more acceptable, though not necessarily when shopping on Fifth Avenue. Other choices include a golf umbrella or a shopping cart. No matter how you disguise it, though, a cane is a hard sell. And yet there is no question that using some kind of support will take pressure off the knee and provide some pain relief. A cane also addresses the unsteadiness some people feel as a result of their pain.

If you've finally given in to using a cane, at least use it correctly! Most people use a cane that is far too long. There should just be a little bend in the elbow. You can't lean as effectively on a cane that's too long. Which hand? You may have heard that for hip problems the cane should be in the hand opposite the painful hip. This is correct. For knees, I leave it to your own discretion.

Braces

Arthritis pain is partly the result of two bones rubbing. A snug brace or tightly wrapped elastic bandage can minimize such rubbing and assuage pain. That is the theory. In my experience, braces and wraps have a low probability of success. With the use of tight wraps, there is the added concern that blood circulation might be compromised. For patients whose arthritis is relatively mild and confined to just the inner aspect of the knee (medial arthritis), there are long leg braces that imperceptibly push the knee into a less bowlegged and more knock-kneed position, thus taking pressure and pain off the inner aspect of the knee. In this specific situation, a brace can be safe and effective, especially if applied to a relatively thin, muscular leg.

Acupuncture

The philosophy of acupuncture is based on the premise that human life flows along fourteen major meridians (channels). Each meridian governs a major organ system. Blockage of a meridian leads to pain or dysfunction, while selective stimulation of meridians restores equilibrium and health. Acupuncture is an accepted adjunct to anesthesia, and I have occasionally seen patients obtain satisfactory relief from acupuncture in the setting of an arthritic knee. As with every other option listed, it is not a cure.

SURGERY

When the time comes for surgery, you can see the glass as being half-full or half-empty. No one likes the idea of having surgery. On the other hand, whereas crutches, walkers, and wheelchairs were the only options available as recently as fifty years ago, today we live in an era in which operations abound.

The best operation for you depends on a number of factors: How much of your knee is arthritic? Which part is arthritic? Are you particularly bowlegged or knock-kneed? Are you athletic? Are you on the younger side or older side? (Under sixty is younger here.) Are you willing to use crutches for three months?

Arthroscopy

This is an outpatient procedure during which the surgeon inserts fine instruments through small puncture holes at the front of the knee (see chapter 3), which allows the knee to be "cleaned out." Imagine a room that is dusty, the upholstery is worn down, and plaster hangs off the ceiling. An arthroscopy cleans the furniture, removes some of that plaster, and perhaps even rearranges the furniture a little. It doesn't reupholster, nor does it replaster. In other words, there is a limit to what an arthroscopy can do. As you may have gathered, the odds of success diminish with the severity of the arthritis. Still, the younger the patient, the lower the threshold for trying an arthroscopy before moving on to a larger operation.

Osteotomy

If you live in the United States, chances are this operation won't be offered to you unless you are quite young. The operation involves cutting the bone and realigning the leg. In the most common scenario, a bowlegged knee is made knock-kneed. The operation is usually recommended to young people whose arthritis is confined to just the inner part of the knee. Crutches are commonly prescribed for three months. An osteotomy has disadvantages: It is somewhat difficult to predict who will obtain a good result.[3] The osteotomy is, in fact, a controlled fracture, and sometimes it does not heal, in which case further surgery is required. Nerves and vessels can be injured during the operation. An osteotomy can make an eventual knee replacement more difficult and less successful. On the other hand, an osteotomy also has several advantages: Assuming that all works out well, you can still participate in any sport you want, and you can also perform heavy labor.

Total Knee Replacement

I never liked this term. It sounds awful. It conjures up the thought of someone whacking out your whole knee. This is not exactly the case. In knee-replacement surgery, the worn-out ends of the bone are removed and replaced with metal on one side and plastic on the other. An analogy can be made with capping a tooth. Or putting in fresh brake pads.

---

3. If you have an academic interest in the subject, you may want to read the following article: R. P. Grelsamer, "Unicompartmental Knee Arthritis—Current Concepts." *J Bone Joint Surg.* 77A (1995): 278–92. Over three hundred references are reviewed in this paper.

> *Total knee replacement* is not a good term. It sounds even more dramatic than it actually is.

Knee replacements are like automobiles to the extent that there exist many models. They have basic similarities and certain differences. New models come out every year. Some have better track records than others. The major distinction between knee replacements and automobiles is that newer cars tend to be better than their predecessors, whereas most new knee replacements land on the trash heap. *No* aspect of medicine or surgery is more carefully hidden from the public than this. It is as big a misconception as there is in the world of orthopedic surgery. The public wants "the latest" implants without realizing what that implies. It means having a knee replacement that will probably not stand the test of time! Without realizing it, the public is literally asking to be experimented on. If you want an implant that will last twenty years, you should ask for one that has been around that long!

Most surgeons do not choose implants based on their track records. Surgeons are easily convinced that the newest implants will solve the imperfections of existing implants, and are therefore easily persuaded to try something new. The orthopedic highway is littered with implants that sounded great initially but then miserably failed. The failures occur years after the surgery. By then the manufacturers have moved on to the next great thing. Surgeons may not be swayed by manufacturers, but they are influenced by surgeons perceived as being leaders in the field. These leaders sometimes have financial ties to the orthopedic manufacturers and are happy to promote new products. To its credit, the orthopedic community demands that speakers and authors reveal their financial ties to the orthopedic industry.

My personal preference for years has been a knee replacement that features a so-called rotating platform. This simple device has been around for twenty years and has an excellent track record. Early on, surgeons predicted that it would not stand the test of time. Now that it has clearly done so, you hear instead that the rotating platform is really unnecessary. Meanwhile, every major orthopedic-implant manufacturer already has a rotating platform implant in the testing phase. I predict that in ten years all surgeons will be using such a product. You heard it here first.

Partial Knee Replacement

In the orthopedic world, they are called "unicompartmental" knee replacements. These small implants replace only the part of the knee that is worn out and are designed for patients whose arthritis is localized to just one part of the knee. Unicompartmental knee replacements are not terribly popular in the United States. They are more difficult to implant than standard knee replacements, and because insurance companies erroneously see them as "half a knee replacement," surgeons get reimbursed half of what they receive for a standard total-knee replacement! Unicompartmental knee replacements are much more popular in the rest of the world, and I suspect that they would be equally popular here if reimbursements were more equitable. I continue to believe that in select patients partial knee replacements are an excellent option.

Cartilage "Growing"

This is a very exciting field. Cartilage normally doesn't grow in the human body. Once it is worn out or injured, it is gone forever. A relatively new concept involves taking cartilage cells from patients, growing them in the laboratory, and reimplant-

Arthritis Treatment Options

Table 5.1

	Pros	Cons	Comments
Medication 1: anti-inflammatory Advil, Motrin, Aleve, Relafen, Naprosyn, Celebrex, Vioxx, etc. Generic: ibuprofen, naproxen	Take away pain without simply masking it	Can cause heartburn or ulcers; possible cartilage damage in the long run	Vary greatly in price
Medication 2: Acetaminophen Tylenol	Few side effects in prescribed doses	Doesn't help solve the underlying problem	Inexpensive
Medication 3: Ultram	Not an anti-inflammatory or a narcotic	Can cause dizziness	
Medication 4: narcotic Tylenol #3, Percocet, Vicodin, Norco	Strong	Addiction, tolerance, drowsiness, constipation	For short-term use only
Physical therapy	No side effects; improves sense of well-being	Time consuming; variable effect	

	Pros	Cons	Comments
Injections 1: Steroids	No effects on stomach; works within a week	Harm to tissues with repeated use	Not the same as taking "steroids" in the athletic sense
Injections 2: Hyaluran (Synvisc, Hyalgan)	"Natural"; rare side effects	Expensive; repeated injections	Work best with mild arthritis
Heat and cold	Soothing; no side effects	Clumsy	Always keep a gel pack around the house
Brace/support	Easy to use	Uncomfortable after a while	Borrow before buying
Cane/stick/umbrella	Surprisingly effective	Yuk	You look old only if you act old
Cushioned shoes	Running shoes are fashionable.	Running shoes aren't that fashionable.	A cushioned insole helps, too.
Nutritional supplements: Glucosamine, Chondroitin sulfate	Harmless for most people	Take a long time to work	Large variations in price for the same products

	Pros	Cons	Comments
Acupuncture	No stomach side effects	Needles	Doesn't cure any more than the other treatments
Weight control	Effective over time	No fun	This is about the only thing under your control!
Water exercises	Stay fit without stressing the knee	Access can be difficult	
Surgery: arthroscopy	Outpatient/low risk	Limited benefit for advanced arthritis	A major surgical advance
Surgery: osteotomy (leg realignment)	No metal or plastic inside the knee	Limited indications	Knock-kneed appearance after surgery
Cartilage growing	The only real "cure" for arthritis	Even more limited indications	Far from perfected; stay tuned
Surgery: knee replacement	Best chance for pain relief: can be total or partial replacement	Inpatient/higher risk than arthroscopy	Another surgical miracle of the twentieth century

ing them in the patient. This is still experimental and is being tried in young patients with very localized arthritis.

Molecular Biology, Genetic Engineering, Stem-Cell Implantation

The future of arthritis therapy lies in these areas. One day, people will view joint replacement surgery the way we quaintly look down upon the crude tools of yesteryear. The injection of that cell or this product will stimulate the body to create fresh cartilage in just the right place. Joint-replacement surgeons will go the way of coopers and swordsmiths. For the moment, though, we have to be grateful for the existence of knee replacements.

DR. G'S TEN-STEP KNEE-ARTHRITIS PROGRAM

Like a man sitting among tin cans without a can opener, a person with knee arthritis can live miserably for lack of a step-by-step guide. Let me take you through a program that has worked well for my patients.

Step 1. Get the Correct Diagnosis

This sounds obvious, but not every painful or creaky knee is arthritic. If you are over sixty years old, chances are that your knee pain is at least in part due to arthritis, but this is not automatic. If you are athletic, you may be suffering from the painful inflammation of one soft tissue or another. For example, the tendon connecting your kneecap to the tibia (shinbone) may be inflamed, and this would be called tendinitis. After a few weeks of living with knee pain, see a health professional to obtain a specific diagnosis. Of course, as oft stated in this book, be leery of the MRI, and be particularly leery of the "torn cartilage" diagnosis.

Step 2. Attitude Adjustment

When given the diagnosis of arthritis, people not uncommonly go through mood swings, especially if they consider themselves to be too young to be tagged with this condition. Denial, anger, and depression are common—a natural reaction to receiving any bad news. Consider the following three case studies:

Fred is fifty-six, and he'll be damned if he's going to modify his lifestyle. He's always jogged on the concrete track near his house, and he regularly hikes the Appalachian trail that runs nearby. Even if it means taking narcotics, he's not going to stop doing the things he loves.

Jane is forty-eight. She had the entire meniscus (cartilage) removed from her knee when she was a teenager, and now she's been told of some early arthritis. She's bummed and feels sorry for herself. She cancels her tennis membership, takes out a subscription to *Modern Maturity*, and ponders her will.

Arthur is fifty-eight. He's been an avid skier, a premier mogul smasher. Regularly lifts weights at the gym. He's just been given the bad news about arthritis in his knee. Upon reflection, he is grateful for the many years of thrilling skiing. Unlike Jane, he doesn't quit. He adapts. He still skis but sticks to the easier runs. At the gym, he's given up the squats, the leg curls, and the "clean and jerks" and has focused more on the abdominals ("abs") and the arms. He has signed up for water aerobics.

Clearly, Arthur has the right attitude. Fred is headed for trouble. When reality sinks in, he'll be that much more depressed. Jane is overreacting. She's letting the diagnosis of arthritis get to her, and she's going to miss out on many enjoyable life experiences. She could still play tennis if she wanted to, but she should back off playing singles on hard courts. She could learn to enjoy doubles and could look into courts with more forgiving surfaces.

When receiving the diagnosis of knee arthritis, you must quickly realize that life is not over. You might need to make some adjustments, but there is no reason why you cannot enjoy life.

Step 3. Over-the-Counter Treatments

Early on, arthritis can be treated with simple remedies. For example, both heat and cold can be soothing, and they have no side effects. I strongly recommend this treatment. Cushioned shoes, such as sneakers and running shoes, take the jarring out of each step. Even so-called city shoes occasionally come with rubber rather than leather soles. I also strongly recommend trying them.

Nutritional supplements, such as glucosamine and chondroitin sulfate, don't have much scientific backing (yet?), but a number of patients report relief from these compounds, and I do recommend them. (Check with your doctor if you are a diabetic. The "glucose" part of glucosamine may or may not be a problem for you.)

Acetaminophen, better known as Tylenol, is a common, inexpensive analgesic that is certainly worth trying. Assuming that you have no stomach problems and are not taking a blood thinner, you can add an over-the-counter anti-inflammatory medication to your regimen. Many people obtain relief with naproxen or ibuprofen (available as generics or as the more expensive Aleve, Advil, Nuprin, or Motrin).

Step 4. Bracing

Wrapping something snuggly around the knee provides relief to many people. This can be in the form of an elastic wrap (Ace, Coban) or a knee support that is slipped on and may be adjusted with straps. It is worth a try. Wear it as much or as little as you like.

Step 5. Exercise

The presence of knee arthritis does not spell the end of exercising. On the contrary. Arthritis tends to cause stiffness, which in turn can lead to greater pain. The stretching and water exercises are strongly advised. In addition to conditioning your knee, these activities will provide you with a sense of well-being.

Step 6. Physical Therapy

A knowledgeable therapist can bring some life back to a painful, stiff knee. In addition to reviewing a stretching program with you, the therapist will provide you with massage and so-called modalities that, well, feel good. Because of the time and expense involved, start with steps 1–5 before going to therapy.

Step 7. Prescription Medications

Once you have been through steps 1–4, you should discuss prescription medications with your doctor. These may have side effects, but they are stronger.

My personal preference is for naproxen, the same medication that is listed in step 3. The prescription version is simply stronger. If you do not tolerate naproxen, many other similar medications are available. If you have a sensitive stomach, the newer COX-2 inhibitors may be for you. They are far more expensive than naproxen and, in my experience, not quite as strong.

Step 8. Use a Hiking Stick or an Umbrella

Leaning on something when you walk takes pressure off the knee. If walking tends to worsen your pain, try a cane. Since canes have a stigma attached to them, consider using a big umbrella or a hiking stick. Some hiking sticks telescope down to a small size, a convenient travel feature.

Step 9. Injections

Injections provide short-term relief. If you are lucky, a steroid injection will be good for a few months. Usually, pain relief lasts from a few days to a few weeks. I therefore recommend steroid injections for people who have a special event coming up. Newer forms of injectable medications may last longer, and they have fewer deleterious effects on the knee. However, their benefits are not predictable, either.

Step 10. Surgery

When all else fails, there is always surgery. Make sure you've tried all else, however!

Fortunately, there are many different kinds of operations available, but keep in mind that there's no minor surgery, only minor surgeons.

Imprecise Radiology Associates

425 Main Street
Anywhere, USA

Jane Smith, MD
13 Central Avenue
Mainstream, USA

    Re: Mr. John Doe

    MRI of the Right Knee

    An MRI of the knee in the axial, sagittal, and coronal images was performed. A joint effusion is noted. The cruciate and collateral complexes are unrevealing. Tear, posterior horn of the medial meniscus is noted. The lateral meniscus is within normal limits. The remainder of the study is unrevealing.

    IMPRESSION:

1. Joint effusion
2. Tear of the posterior horn of the medial meniscus

B.S., MD
Board Certified Radiologist

Fig. 5.3. Misleading MRI report in a patient with severe arthritis. Note the ubiquitous "torn meniscus." There is no mention of the patient's most pressing problem: very severe arthritis. Note that this arthritis was already very clear on the thirty-dollar X ray called the "Merchant view." The MRI in this patient was unnecessary, poorly read, and misleading.

Chapter 6

The Hidden Causes of Knee Pain, Part I

*I*F YOU RISE AWKWARDLY FROM A KNEELING POSITION AND TEAR a cartilage in your knee, the diagnosis will be obvious to any practitioner. Not all conditions, however, are so clear. Somewhere between the domains of the obvious and the unsolvable lie well-described conditions that elude the average provider of knee care. These I term the "hidden causes" of knee pain. We will start with what, in my practice, has been one of the largest causes of "mysterious" pain.

What's Wrong With This Picture?

Sally M. is thirty-four years old. She was fine until she fell and landed on her left knee four years ago. She had an MRI within a week of the injury and was told she had a torn cartilage. She had physical therapy that consisted of an exercise bicycle and "funny pads" placed around her knee. Six weeks after her injury, she underwent an arthroscopy, after which she felt no better. She went for more sessions of exercise on the bicycle until her insurance refused to pay for more therapy. She tried various anti-inflammatory medications and started to take narcotics. Her friends and employer started to think she was perhaps looking for sympathy. She was sent for a psychological evaluation. It was recommended that perhaps she needed another MRI and another arthroscopy to remove scar tissue from the first operation.

The above scenario is more common than you might imagine. There are many things wrong with this picture, some of which you probably recognize from reading the previous chapters.

1. Most of the time it is unreasonable to obtain an MRI soon after a simple injury: It is not likely to affect the treatment, it can miss important conditions, and conversely, the MRI may be "overread" as showing torn cartilage.
2. The finding of a torn cartilage in someone who has bumped his or her knee is likely to be either wrong or irrelevant.
3. Surgery for a torn cartilage in this setting is therefore doomed to failure right from the start.
4. Finally, simply using an exercise bicycle, putting weights on your ankle, and getting a little electrical stimulation are simply not adequate physical therapy for a number of knee conditions.

Many patients present to my office with persistent knee pain. They have already seen other doctors, they have all had expensive tests, and many have already had one or more operations. Yet they still have pain. Some are worse than they were originally. This is partly explained by the fact that many conditions will not show up on routine testing, testing that doctors rely on excessively to make a diagnosis. For example, as doctors squeeze more and more patients into their schedule, the MRI instead of the doctor increasingly "makes" the diagnosis. The doctor listens to you for a few seconds, puts his hands on your knee for a few more moments, and then waits for the MRI to tell you what your diagnosis is. By this point in the book, we've discussed at length what the problem is with that approach, but it bears repeating one more time. Finding the cause of knee pain by obtaining an MRI is equivalent to judging today's temperature by looking at a satellite picture: It would be an expensive way to do things, and it might still not give you the requisite information!

> Kneecap conditions are among the most misdiagnosed in all of medicine.

KNEECAP MALALIGNMENT

In my experience, kneecap malalignment represents the *greatest* area of misdiagnosis of the knee. It is a field that is very poorly appreciated by orthopedists, physical therapists, rheumatologists, radiologists, physiatrists (rehabilitation specialists), chiropractors, and other health professionals dealing with knee pain.

Basic Anatomy

The kneecap sits in a groove called the trochlea, or trochlear groove (fig. 6.1). On occasion, the groove is shallow or flat or even inverted. In other words, it is possible for the groove to be convex, like a fried egg, in which case the kneecap/trochlea construct is highly unstable.

There are four muscles connected to the upper part of the kneecap; collectively, these are called the quadriceps (literally, four heads). They include the rectus femoris, the vastus intermedius, the vastus lateralis, and the vastus medialis.

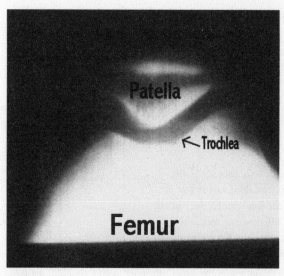

Fig. 6.1. The so-called patellofemoral joint. *Patella* is the medical term for kneecap. It is the bone that sits at the front of the knee. Roundish when seen from the front, it is triangular in cross section. It slides up and down in a groove at the end of the femur (thighbone) called the *trochlea*.

The name "quadriceps" comes from the fact that there are four (quad) muscles. They are all attached to the kneecap.

All tend to pull the kneecap toward the head, but whereas the first two pull straight up, the vastus lateralis pulls the kneecap up and out, so to speak, and the vastus medialis pulls up and in (see fig. 6.2). The kneecap is connected to the rectus femoris and to the vastus intermedius via a broad, flat tendon called the quadriceps tendon. At the other end, the kneecap is attached to the tibia by way of the patellar tendon, occasionally called the patellar ligament.[1] The net result of all these connections is a straightening of the knee when the quadriceps muscles contract.

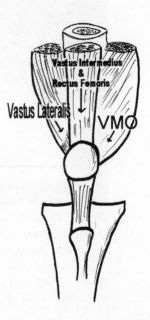

Fig. 6.2. The muscles of the quadriceps. The vastus lateralis pulls the kneecap to the outside; the VMO (vastus medialis obliquus) pulls the kneecap to the inside. The rectus femoris and vastus intermedius tend to pull the kneecap straight up.

---

1. Bands of tissue connecting one bone to another are called *ligaments,* while bands of tissue connecting muscles to bone are called *tendons.* Since the biological rope we are discussing connects the kneecap to the shinbone, in one sense it is a ligament. On the other hand, functionally speaking, this rope is but a continuation of the quadriceps muscles (and of the quadriceps tendon). In this sense, our rope is a tendon; thus, the term *patellar tendon.*

In more ways than one, the kneecap mechanism, anatomically speaking, "rounds a corner." Not only is the kneecap draped over the end of the thighbone like a waterfall, but when seen from the front, the quadriceps, kneecap, and patellar tendon form a sharp angle (see fig. 6.3). In some people, this angle (called the quadriceps, or "Q" angle) is particularly pronounced, and it contributes to the overall malalignment of the kneecap. Because of this unique setup, every time the quadriceps muscles contract, the kneecap tends to be pulled to the outside part of the knee. This is termed the bowstring effect.

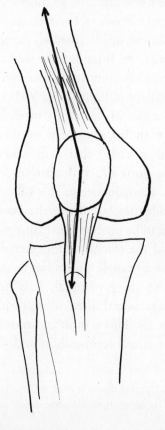

Fig. 6.3. The quadriceps muscle and tendon form an angle called the Q angle. When this angle is pronounced, the kneecap tends to be pulled out of its groove.

The outside (lateral) wall of the trochlear groove is higher than the inside (medial) wall. When all is well, this helps to counter the bowstring effect.

> Kneecap malalignment is associated with a number of possible anatomic variations.

There are other parts of the anatomy that either exacerbate or counter the bowstring effect. For example, the "lateral retinaculum" is a tough, broad band of tissue attached to the entire outside (lateral) part of the kneecap.[2] Predictably, it tends to pull the kneecap to the outside. On the inside (medial) aspect of the kneecap lies the medial retinaculum. It tends to be weaker than its lateral counterpart and receives significant assistance from a muscle called the vastus medialis obliquus (aka VMO). The VMO is actually the lower portion of the vastus medialis that we discussed above. People with malalignment of their kneecap are commonly cursed with a VMO that is deficient: The fibers are too vertical, and they don't attach themselves far enough down on the kneecap. The consequence of this suboptimal setup is a VMO that does adequately balance the bowstring effect. This leads the kneecap to be pushed up against the lateral wall of the trochlea or out of the trochlea altogether. In cross section, the kneecap looks like a triangle. It lies flat in the trochlea. In other words, relative to the horizontal, it is not tilted. In some patients, however, it is indeed tilted, always with the "lateral" side down (fig. 6.4 A & B). This is most commonly associated with an excessively tight lateral retinaculum and, in

---

2. Lateral means away from the midline; medial means toward the midline. Thus, the little toe is lateral to the big toe, and the big toe is medial to the second toe.

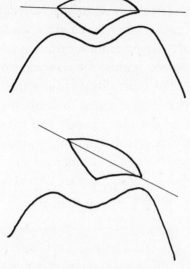

Fig. 6.4A. The normal kneecap sits flush within the trochlear groove.

Fig. 6.4B. In some people, it is tilted.

my experience, is the most common form of kneecap malalignment. Whether the tight lateral retinaculum is the cause or the result of the tilt remains a subject of debate.

The cartilaginous underbelly of the kneecap features "facets," that is, angled surfaces. If the doctor palpates these facets by curling his fingers around the kneecap, this should not be painful. This maneuver, on the other hand, is painful in patients whose kneecaps are poorly aligned.[3]

The combination of tilt and tender facets is, in my opinion, evidence that part of your problem is the kneecap. It's that simple.

You should know that this is not a universal truth. Otherwise knowledgeable health professionals state that tilted kneecaps are normal, and they base that argument on the fact

---

3. Cartilage itself has no nerve fibers and cannot register pain. The underlying bone, however, is richly innervated and very sensitive to pain.

that they often see tilted kneecaps that are painless. It is my feeling that they are confusing the term *normal* in the everyday sense of the word with "normal" as it might be used in the world of medicine. "Normal" in everyday language means common or acceptable. In that sense, it is indeed normal for a segment of the population to develop cancer or heart disease. But a medically normal condition is one that does not lead to death, disease, or pain, and in that sense of the word, cancer and heart disease are clearly not normal. Kneecap malalignment is normal in the "common" sense of the word but not in the medical sense. An analogy here can be made with flat feet: They are common, they are not necessarily painful, but they are not normal.

> Some doctors still refer to kneecap problems as "chondromalacia."

The kneecap serves a number of important functions: Most significantly, it is a complex lever that provides a mechanical advantage to the thigh muscles. Without a kneecap, your quadriceps muscles (at the front of the thigh) have to work harder. This is what happens when the kneecap is surgically removed, and it is not a procedure I commonly recommend. Although some patients can compensate for this kneecap absence, others develop muscle fatigue and/or arthritis from the increased stress on the rest of the knee.

As the knee bends and straightens, the kneecap glides in a groove located at the end of the thighbone (fig. 6.5). Roughly speaking, the undersurface of the kneecap looks like a *U,* and it matches the *U* shape of the groove. There are a number of potential problems here: In some people the fit is rather loose, and the kneecap slips in and out. This leads to a sensation of the

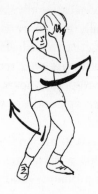

Fig. 6.5. Twisting the upper body while keeping the feet planted on the ground can force the kneecap to slip out of its groove. This occurs most commonly with dancing and basketball.

knee giving out (fig. 6.5). In other patients the kneecap may stay in the groove and yet be poorly positioned ("malaligned")—much as the wheel on a car might be out of alignment. This can be painful because one side of the kneecap does all the work and starts to get sore.

If your knee slips out of its groove, there is a reasonable chance that the correct diagnosis will be made. Even so, many an unstable kneecap has been mistaken for a torn ligament. If, however, your knee simply hurts because of malalignment, chances are that it will be completely missed by the person looking after you.

> Kneecap conditions are underdiagnosed and over-operated!

Considering the number of excellent doctors around and how common kneecap problems are, you probably wonder how it could be possible for the condition to be so frequently misdiagnosed. The answer lies in the erratic dissemination of medical knowledge. A new concept or treatment may occasionally sweep over the medical community (e.g., Viagra!), but more commonly, it gradually seeps into everyday practice, a little faster here, a little slower there. Kneecap conditions are well recognized in certain parts of the world and more poorly acknowledged in others. Strange as it may seem, kneecap conditions are relatively unappreciated in the United States.

Kneecap problems mimic other knee conditions. In 1940, Dr. Karlsson in Sweden noted that surgeons were taking out torn cartilage for what was really a kneecap problem—and this was in 1940, when removing a cartilage was a serious endeavor (a large scar and five days in the hospital). Nowadays, removing a meniscus is a relatively small outpatient procedure that neither doctors nor patients think twice about. The problem of "mistaken identity" has therefore been hugely magnified! Europeans are not the only ones who have picked up on the problem: Jack Hughston, a remarkably famous orthopedist from our very own country, noted as far back as 1960 that "the orthopaedic surgeon who has not mistaken a recurrent subluxation of the patella for a torn medial meniscus has undoubtedly had a very limited and fortunate experience with knees and meniscectomies." And yet the message has been painfully slow to get through to the rank and file. A large percentage of patients with knee pain get a (needless) MRI, a large percentage of those MRIs are (erroneously) read as showing a torn cartilage, and a large percentage of these patients are scheduled for unnecessary surgery.

In the United States, orthopedists are not rescued by radiologists. Radiologists detect fractures, arthritis, and various bone diseases that the orthopedist might not have suspected. But when it comes to the kneecap, the radiologist is likely to know even less than the orthopedist. Even when an abnormality exists with respect to the patella, the X-ray report is likely to simply read "no fracture, no dislocation." This is technically correct: There is no fracture, and crudely speaking, everything appears in place. But the fact that the kneecap might by lying too high or too tilted is altogether omitted. The simplest views of the knee are called the "AP" and the "lateral." The AP is the front-to-back view; the lateral is the side view. If the lateral is carried out just right, a great deal of information can be obtained about the kneecap and its underlying groove. An additional view, called the Merchant view (named after Alan Merchant, M.D., from California), provides yet further information. For this view, you lie on your back with your legs off the X-ray table and resting on a special device that maintains your knees bent any-where from 30 degrees (ideally) to 45 degrees (see chapter 8). This view should be obtained in anyone who could conceivably have a kneecap problem or with suspect findings on a well-executed lateral view.

> Kneecap malalignment is often detected on a good set of plain X rays!

The Perfect Crime

The innocent patient presents to the doctor with knee pain. Using a misleading MRI (see fig. 6.9), the surgeon sells an op-eration to the patient. The surgeon informs the patient that it may take a few weeks for the full effects of the surgery to be ap-parent. (This is actually true.) After surgery, the patient goes for physical therapy and does eventually get better. The surgeon has earned a few dollars, the patient is thrilled with her surgeon, everybody's happy, and there's no problem, right? Wrong. You've just witnessed the perfect crime. With time and appropriate physical therapy the patient was going to get better, anyway! Who is ever going to know? This is a victimless crime. These useless operations lead to some increase in our insurance premiums, but who is going to notice? There is another catch, though: There is no risk-free surgery. Even with a "minor" procedure such as an arthroscopy, some patients fail to get better or, worse yet, develop complications. This, then, is my main objection to gratuitous knee surgery.

Making the Right Diagnosis

One of the first things they teach you in medical school is that you can't make a diagnosis you haven't thought of. Therefore, the right diagnosis will never be made if the doctor isn't at least considering your kneecap as a potential problem. The diagnosis of kneecap malalignment is made on the physical examination and can often be confirmed on routine X rays or MRI. Therein lies another problem: The doctor has to actually take the time to examine you thoroughly. If he wants to confirm the diagnosis on an X ray, he has to be particularly adept at ordering and reading those special views. Should he wish confirmation on an MRI, he has to make sure that the MRI is complete (see fig. 6.9) and that either he or the radiologist is familiar with the interpretation of kneecap problems on MRIs. In my experience, these conditions are not always met.

Treatment

The Kneecap "Cure"

While making the diagnosis can be difficult, the treatment is surprisingly straightforward (see table 6.1); 95 percent of patients improve with a nonoperative program, the cornerstone of which is appropriate physical therapy. The key word here is appropriate. Twenty minutes on an exercise bicycle, a few warm towels, and electrical stimulation with those funny little pads do not constitute an appropriate program for this condition. It is upsetting to me to find people scheduled for surgery on the basis of "failed physical therapy" when in fact they never had suitable therapy to begin with.

> Physical therapy has to be carried out by a particularly knowledgeable person.

Therapy for this condition includes *stretching* of the major muscle groups about the knee. This includes the hamstrings at the back of your thigh, the quadriceps muscles at the front of your thigh, the adductor muscles at the inner thigh, and the iliotibial band that runs along the outer part of the thigh. You can perform some of these exercises at home. In fact, you should. It's like learning the piano: Practice between the lessons! Through skillful manipulation, the therapist may also gradually stretch the lateral retinaculum (see "Basic Anatomy," page 108).

Taping is a technique whereby special tape is applied to the front of the knee. It is applied in such a way as to pull the skin in one direction or another. Because the kneecap is (loosely) connected to the skin, the kneecap is pulled along in the direction of the skin. Thus, pull the kneecap toward a more normal position. This at least is the theory. The extent to which this really takes place remains a subject of controversy. But the fact that a number of patients with malalignment are helped by this approach is, in my experience, unequivocal. Some people learn the technique from their therapist and tape their knee at home.

There have even been reports of salacious taping parties at the White House! (Just seeing if you're paying attention.)

Biofeedback and surface electromyography are more sophisticated (less accessible) physical-therapy modalities that help the patient monitor progress. Most important of all, physical therapy for kneecap conditions requires significant attention on the part of the therapy team. Not all therapy outfits are geared for that approach. Unfortunately, in a managed-care setting it is true that this kind of attention may not be cost-effective (for the therapist).

Surgery

In case you've zoomed right to this section, keep in mind that it is the rare patient with kneecap problems who needs surgery. If you need surgery, it's either because you've failed a thorough nonoperative program, your malalignment is truly severe, or your kneecap is very arthritic.

Compared to surgery for other conditions, surgery for kneecap problems is less rewarding, and choosing the right operation is a major source of debate at orthopedic meetings. Over 150 procedures have been described through the years, and there are currently dozens of procedures still in use. There are two camps: (1) surgeons who perform an outpatient (small-incision) procedure first and then come back later for a bigger procedure if necessary; (2) surgeons who perform the definitive procedure from the start if they feel that the small procedure has a low chance of success. By and large I am in the second camp. Patients are not usually grateful for an operation that doesn't work, even if it is a small operation. They are even less grateful when they discover that the "small" operation isn't always so small when it comes to recovery and complications. In select cases, however, I am amenable to first trying the smaller procedure.

For patients whose kneecap slips in and out of the groove, the challenge for the surgeon is to tighten the kneecap without tightening it so much that arthritis will develop in later years. At least one operation has become notorious for this complication.[4] In patients whose main complaint is pain, the challenge is simply to provide lasting pain relief.

Kneecap operations can be divided into those that realign the kneecap and those that do not. Realignment operations are by and large performed when the kneecap is felt to be out of place. These operations can also be performed if the cartilage under the kneecap is unhealthy and if the surgeon feels that moving the kneecap one way or the other might take pressure off these unhealthy areas.

The orthopedic community distinguishes between proximal and distal realignment operations. The word *proximal* means close to the center of the body; *distal* means far from it. Thus, in orthopedic lingo, the ankle would be distal to the knee, the hip would be proximal to the knee, etc. Proximal procedures involve surgery on the tissues that surround the kneecap, while distal realignments are performed farther down on the "tibial tuberosity"—the bump at the top of the tibia (shinbone) where the kneecap ligament attaches itself (see fig. 6.6).

The following is a thumbnail summary of some the operations you're likely to hear about.

Proximal realignments include:

• *The lateral retinacular release (commonly abbreviated "lateral release").* When the lateral retinaculum is tight, it tugs on the kneecap. The kneecap becomes tilted like a beret and/or pulled off to the side. The concept of the lateral release is therefore sim-

---

4. The Hauser procedure, which was developed in the 1930s by Emil Hauser, from Chicago.

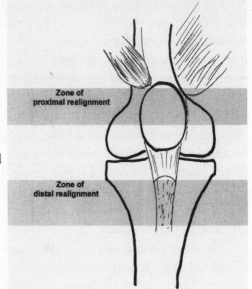

Fig. 6.6. Operations that realign the kneecap are divided into proximal and distal procedures.

ple. As described in the 1970s by Ficat in France and by Merchant in the United States, the lateral retinaculum is cut as it inserts onto the kneecap and the kneecap tendon. It was a brilliant idea that was rapidly embraced by the orthopedic community. The concept of an unstable kneecap is as ancient as human civilization, but until the 1970s no one had thought that a tilted kneecap could be painful. That a relatively simple procedure could cure this heretofore mysterious kneecap pain made the operation deliciously enticing. The procedure became that much more appealing in the 1980s when it was discovered that the release could be carried out via a small incision or even arthroscopically (without incisions or scars): The surgeon visualizes the inside of the knee through an arthroscope.[5] He or she

5. The arthroscope is a pencil-like instrument introduced into a joint via a small hole (see chapter 3).

then cuts the lateral retinaculum from the inside of the knee, proceeding up to—but not through—the skin. The lateral release became wildly popular, and surgeons began to expand the indications for this procedure to anybody with unexplained knee pain. It was too good to be true.

> Because a partial lateral release can be carried out arthroscopically without a scar, it is vastly overused.

And it was. Results started to come in. In the first place, the lateral release is not completely innocuous. Coursing through the lateral retinaculum is a group of blood vessels that readily bleed when cut. These are the "geniculate" vessels. They are quite pernicious to the extent that, when cut, they may not bleed right away. Instead, they go into spasm. This stops the bleeding. At least temporarily. Within a short time—but after the patient has left the operating room—the spasm resolves. The geniculates begin to bleed. The knee swells as it fills with blood. This is painful and limits the patient's knee motion. At the first postoperative visit the surgeon has to "tap" the knee, that is, place a needle into the joint to draw out the blood. Doing so is not a major crowd pleaser. Moreover, even though the lateral release leaves little or no traces, it is still an operation. It is therefore subject to all the potential complications of an operation, including infections and RSD (see chapter 7). Such complications are rare. Less rare is the very real "complication" of not making the patient feel any better.

There are a number of reasons why a lateral release, by itself, may not work. In the first place, the operation is rarely performed as it was first described. Instead of extending from the top of the kneecap down to the tibial tuberosity (at the top of the shin), most lateral releases go only half that distance for that's as far as you can go with a small incision or with an arthroscopy. (The original operation involved a significant incision down the middle of the knee.) Therefore, the release as it is performed today is incomplete relative to the original version. The kneecap is consequently not released as much. Why not do it the original way? Orthopedically speaking, it is politically incorrect to offer a lateral release through a longish incision down the center of the knee. Offered this way in the new millennium, the lateral release would send the potential patient scampering to another surgeon, who would gladly offer to perform the procedure arthroscopically. The arthroscopic procedure is nearly irresistible to the unwary patient. The original (first-opinion) surgeon simply looks old-fashioned.

A second limitation of the lateral release is that it does not predictably correct all that is wrong: In the same way that a lateral retinaculum might be tight, the medial retinaculum might be lax, and the VMO muscle can be deficient. The Q angle is occasionally very elevated, and arthritic lesions may be present under the kneecap or in the trochlea. The kneecap can lie too high (patella alta) or too low (patella baja, aka infera). The trochlea can be convex instead of concave. With the exception of very specific arthritic lesions, the lateral release is not going to address these deficiencies.

At the present time, the role of the isolated lateral release is a hotly contested issue in the world of orthopedics.

• *The medial plication/VMO advancement.* As previously noted, the medial retinaculum and VMO can be deficient. To address this, the medial retinaculum is detached from the kneecap and then reattached over the kneecap. Alternatively, a portion of the retinaculum is removed, and the remainder is reattached to the side of the kneecap, whence it came. Either way, the kneecap is pulled medially (toward the inside). The

VMO can be detached from the quadriceps tendon and from the upper medial corner of the kneecap and pulled down in the direction of its fibers onto the kneecap. Again, the effect is to pull the kneecap over medially.[6] This operation is usually performed in combination with a lateral release and therefore requires a separate incision. The alternative is an incision down the middle of the knee, which gives the surgeon access to both sides of the kneecap.

• *Denervation.* By cutting through both the medial and lateral retinaculum, the surgeon interrupts a significant percentage of the nerves that transmit pain from the kneecap. Cynics will say that the above-mentioned operations relieve pain not because the kneecap has been realigned but because the sensory-nerve supply has been interrupted. There may be some truth to this. But not enough truth to make it a completely reliable approach.

Distal realignments include:

• *Moving the tibial tuberosity medially (to the inside; fig. 6.7).* This goes by different names around the world. In the United States it is called the Elmslie-Trillat operation. Some surgeons have used this operation routinely for patients whose kneecaps slip out of the trochlear groove. It cannot be used in children with much growth left, as it can harm part of the growth plate in the shinbone.

No other orthopedic condition is associated with so many different operations.

6. And posteriorly, if overdone.

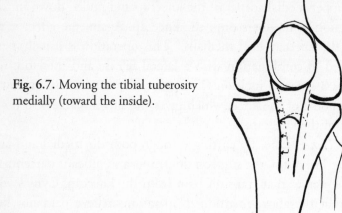

Fig. 6.7. Moving the tibial tuberosity medially (toward the inside).

Because an abnormal position of the tibial tuberosity leads to an elevated Q angle (see above), the least controversial indication for the Elmslie-Trillat operation is an elevated Q angle. The most controversial aspect of the operation is its use in patients whose tibial tuberosity is normally positioned to begin with.

When the tibial tuberosity is moved to its new position, it needs to be fixed with one or two screws, and the patient has to limit his or her activities for six to twelve weeks, until the tuberosity has healed in its new position. Depending on how solidly fixed these screws are, a cast or soft knee immobilizer will be used until the tuberosity has sufficiently healed.

• *The Maquet.* This tibial-tuberosity operation is named after the Belgian surgeon who first described it. As of this writing, it has lost much of its popularity in Europe, but it remains an accepted procedure. It is designed to lift the kneecap out of the trochlear groove, thus taking pressure off it. Unfortunately, it mostly lifts the nose ("distal pole") of the kneecap and does

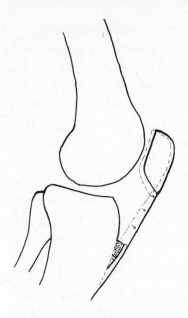

Fig. 6.8. The Maquet operation elevates the tibial tuberosity (brings it forward). It thereby lifts part of the kneecap off the femur (thighbone).

not predictably relieve pain. To carry out the operation, the tibial tuberosity is partially split off from the underlying shinbone, and a piece of bone is inserted between the shinbone and the tuberosity (fig. 6.8). This elevates the tuberosity. Since the patellar tendon inserts itself onto the tuberosity, the tendon is elevated, and since the tendon starts at the tip of the kneecap, the tip of the kneecap is elevated. Just how much to elevate the tuberosity, where the bone should come from, what bone substitutes are acceptable, how the Maquet procedure should be fixed (screws?) until it heals, and what currently should be the indications of the operation are just some of the controversies surrounding it.

• *The Fulkerson (AMZ).* This is a combination of the two tibial-tuberosity transfers described above. The tuberosity is both elevated and transposed medially (to the inside) through a single oblique cut between the tuberosity and the underlying bone. John Fulkerson, M.D., has popularized it in the United

States. He has called the procedure an "anteromedialization" of the tuberosity and has abbreviated it AMZ. It combines the advantages and disadvantages of the Elmslie-Trillat and the Maquet and is therefore equally controversial. My personal indication for this operation is a patient who, in my opinion, would benefit from both the Elmslie-Trillat and the Maquet.

• *The distal transfer.* If the kneecap sits too high in the groove (patella alta), the tibial tuberosity can be brought distally (down toward the foot) by one or two centimeters. The procedure is less commonly performed in the United States than the above-mentioned operations in part because severe patella alta is relatively uncommon and is underrecognized in the United States (see chapters 2 and 8).

Note: The distal realignments can all be performed with any of the proximal realignments. This makes for an impressive combination of surgical permutations. The knowledgeable surgeon will think this through carefully and do his best to put together the combination that's right for you.

KNEECAP ARTHRITIS

Sometimes putting the kneecap where it belongs is not enough. If arthritis already exists under the kneecap or in the underlying trochlear groove, one can still have pain even if the kneecap is in the correct position. Assuming you've tried and failed the arthritis treatment choices listed in chapter 5, the surgeon now has the following options: He or she can move the kneecap up, down, left, or right in such a way as to take pressure off the raw area(s). This is only an alternative if most of the cartilage is intact.

Other options include taking cartilage plugs from a different part of the knee to replace the worn area (similar to the hairplug technique). It has not worked well for arthritis about the kneecap. Alternatively, a small amount of cartilage can be harvested from another part of the knee; sent to a laboratory, which "cultures" the cartilage until it has grown to the size of a thimble; and reintroduced into the knee and placed into the raw, arthritic areas. This technique has demonstrated reasonable results in other parts of the knee, but the statistics are less encouraging around the kneecap. The raw surfaces can be carefully hammered with a sharp object in order to create punctate holes through the hard, underlying bone. This brings blood to the surface and with it, one hopes, cartilage-producing cells. This is not a predictable technique, but it is relatively void of complications. In its various incarnations, the operation has been called the Pridie technique and, more recently, the microfracture technique.

The worn undersurface of the kneecap can be replaced with a plastic implant, while the trochlear groove is covered with a fine, metallic shield—in effect, a partial knee replacement, with many of the pros and cons associated with joint-replacement surgery (see chapter 5). A complete knee replacement is always an option, as it is for any arthritis anywhere in the knee.

As a final choice, the kneecap can be removed outright, which is called a patellectomy. Although some patients do quite well with this approach, the kneecap serves a useful function for most people (see "Kneecap Malalignment" at the beginning of this chapter). As of this writing there is no turning back once the kneecap has been removed. It is also not 100 percent predictable with regard to pain relief, especially if arthritis is also present in the trochlear groove.

CHONDROMALACIA

If you're familiar with this word, you might wonder how it fits in with this section. I have studiously avoided using it, for *chon-*

dromalacia is a treacherous term. It means many things to many people, including pain in the front of the knee, pain from kneecap malalignment, cartilage damage under the kneecap, cartilage damage anywhere in the knee, or arthritis. Gradually, the term is being abandoned, though not fast enough. Over the last fifty years chondromalacia has become an accepted expression, and in the United States there is even an insurance code for it (717.7). If your pain is toward the front of the knee and the doctor can't find much wrong, he will in all likelihood tell you that you are suffering from chondromalacia.[7] Thus, kneecap problems are also overdiagnosed!

In short, kneecap problems are misdiagnosed in both directions: Patients are told that they have chondromalacia when in fact there is not much wrong with their kneecap, and conversely, when they truly have painful kneecap malalignment there is a good chance that it will be missed.

7. Unfortunately, if there is anything wrong with your articular cartilage (see chapter 5), it will also be labeled chondromalacia, which can lead to tremendous confusion.

The Nonoperative Treatment of Patellar Pain

Table 6.1

Treatment	Pros	Cons
Activity modification	Works to some extent	Are you willing to give up that sport?
Physical therapy	Usually helps	Needs to be supervised by a very knowledge-able person
Home exercises	Effective in maintaining what's been taught in physical therapy	Boring
Brace	Few side effects	Trial and error to find the right one
Anti-inflammatory medication	Quiets pain by diminishing inflammation	Can't take pills forever
Analgesic (e.g., acetaminophen)	Few stomach side effects	Limited effect
Cold/heat	Quiets pain without "pills"	Mainly useful at home; cumbersome
Injections	Work in the short run	Limited effect. Who wants injections?
Weight reduction	Takes a great deal of pressure off the kneecap	Takes a great deal of self-discipline

Incomplete Imaging
525 Main Street
Anywhere, USA

Joan Jones, MD
25 Main Drive
Anywhere, United States of America

Patient: Mary Smith
Study: MRI Left Knee

Images were obtained in the sagittal plane using a T1 weighted pulse and T2 weighted pulse sequences. Coronal T1 weighted images were also obtained.

Osseous structures are grossly intact.

The anterior and posterior cruciate ligaments are preserved. A Grade I signal is noted in the medial collateral ligament (MCL). The extensor mechanism is intact.

A Grade II tear is found in the posterior horn of the medial meniscus. There is no tear of the lateral meniscus.

A small suprapatellar joint effusion is noted. A Baker's cyst is also noted.

Impression: •   Grade II tear of the posterior horn of the medial meniscus.
•   Grade I tear of the MCL.
•   Joint effusion.
•   Baker's cyst

Fig. 6.9. A misleading MRI report in a patient with kneecap pain.

Note the inaccurate or irrelevant findings. I count at least five of them.

1. The so-called grade II tear of the meniscus is not a tear. It represents a chemical change within the meniscus (cartilage), it is not visible to the naked eye, and it does not cause knee pain.

2. An injury is required to tear the medial collateral ligament (MCL). This patient had no injury. The "grade I" tear seen by the radiologist therefore represents a slight variation in the composition of the ligament and does not shed light on the patient's condition.

3. *Joint effusion* means *water on the knee.* This is found in just about any patient whose knee is irritated for whatever reason. In and of itself, it is not painful, and its presence does not help the doctor diagnose the source of the pain.

4. The Baker's cyst is a pouch at the back of the knee. Normal joint fluid sometimes collects in that pouch. It is a common finding, and it is not painful.

5. The radiologist proceeds to omit the most glaring problem: The patient has a serious disorder of the kneecap and of the underlying groove. The reason for the omission is simple: The MRI is incomplete. Note in the first line of the report that only sagittal and coronal views were taken. A third set of views, called "axial" views, are required to completely judge the position of the kneecap. These views are carried out in good MRI facilities.

Chapter 7

The Hidden Causes of Knee Pain, Part II

A NUMBER OF PAINFUL KNEE CONDITIONS WILL ESCAPE DETEC-
tion if the treating doctor relies solely on the MRI to make a diagnosis. In chapter 6 we reviewed the large subject of pain
pertaining to malalignment of the kneecap. In this chapter, we
will discuss equally painful and equally "hidden" sources of knee
pain.

TIGHTNESS OF THE ITB AND RUNNER'S KNEE

ITB stands for iliotibial band. This tough strap of tissue runs
from the outer aspect of the upper leg, down the outside of the
thigh, across the knee joint, and into the upper tibia, or shinbone (fig. 7.1). It fulfills a remarkable number of functions, one

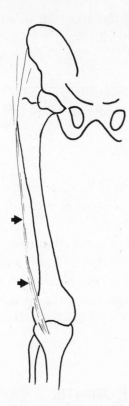

Fig. 7.1. The iliotibial band (ITB) runs down the outer aspect of the leg. When excessively tight, it can cause knee pain.

of which is to keep you from looking bowlegged every time you take a step. It is also happens to be connected to your kneecap. The ITB is prone to tightness for reasons that remain unclear, and when this happens, a number of painful possibilities may ensue: For example, the ITB can rub against the side of the femur (thighbone), giving rise to "runner's knee" (see page 136). The ITB can also pull the kneecap off to the side, leading to painfully abnormal pressures about the kneecap.

The diagnosis of a tight ITB is easy to make. The patient's legs are positioned in a certain manner, and the doctor notes whether or not the upper leg can be lowered to the examination table. This is called the Ober test. If the upper leg fails to fall down onto the table, the ITB is too tight.

> Many painful conditions will not show up on an MRI!

Most patients with a painfully tight ITB can be treated with a stretching program supervised by a physical therapist. But someone has to have made the diagnosis!

All too often, the doctor skips these time-consuming little tests and goes right for the MRI. *But a tight ITB does not show up on an MRI!* What shows up instead is the ubiquitous reading of a torn meniscus, and, yes, here we go again, the doctor may recommend surgery.

RUNNER'S KNEE / TENDINITIS

There are tendons everywhere about the knee, and they can become irritated, which is painful. The pain can be associated with bending and straightening the knee, and if the condition is severe enough, the pain can even be present at rest. Usually, the diagnosis can be made by palpation of the painful area. Again, this requires some attention on the part of the examining physician. Note once more that tendinitis of the knee does not routinely show up on an MRI! You will therefore be misdiagnosed by any practitioner who relies extensively on the MRI.

The most common tendons to become irritated are the iliotibial band (ITB) and the patellar tendon.

Runner's Knee

Runner's knee is the name given to an inflammation of the lower part of the ITB just as it crosses the upper part of the knee. In the susceptible person, it comes from repeatedly bending the knee back and forth. It happens most commonly in runners, but just as tennis elbow doesn't happen only to tennis players, runner's knee can happen to cyclists, soccer players, lacrosse players, in fact, to just about any athlete who runs. The pain is localized in the lowermost part of the outer thigh, right over the knobby part of the knee. Typically, the pain doesn't kick in until the runner has reached a certain mileage ("Doc, I'm fine until I reach 2.5 miles"), and it subsides with rest. It also hurts when you press right over the outer aspect of the knee. If you suspect that's what you are suffering from, try an ITB stretching program (see figure 11.6), make sure you've warmed up before running, and for two weeks or so, consider taking an over-the-counter anti-inflammatory medication, such as ibuprofen or naproxen, prior to running. If your knee still hurts when you come home from running, applying a cold pack to the painful area can reduce the pain. When running, temporarily cut back to mileage that doesn't hurt. Or switch to swimming for a week or two if you can. Then gradually work up the mileage. I haven't found braces to be particularly useful for runner's knee, but if a friend of yours has one, try it. It won't do you any harm. Avoid running along the side of the hill (it makes you run crooked) and make sure your shoes aren't worn down. In fact, think back to whether your pain started when you bought your latest running shoes. Every shoe turns your foot in an ever so slightly different way, and sometimes that's enough to throw off your knee mechanics. So if the start of your pain coincided with your latest shoe purchase, try a model that resembles your old shoes. Are you flat-footed? Are your arches high? Think about a consultation with a podiatrist for full-length shoe orthotics (devices you slip into a shoe). When all else fails, buy some new clothing. Seems to work for my wife.

Patellar Tendinitis

The patellar tendon connects the kneecap (patella) to the tibia (shinbone). It can become irritated in athletes who repeatedly jump. The pain and tenderness are localized in the lower part of the kneecap or in the area just below. Treatment involves (yikes!) holding off on that basketball playing until things quiet down. As with any tendinitis, adjunctive management includes anti-inflammatory medication and physical therapy (the application of ultrasound and related treatments). If the tendinitis is so severe that it interferes with everyday activities, you may need a brace that doesn't let you bend the knee: a knee immobilizer. Indeed, every time you bend the knee, you are tugging on the kneecap and on the tendon connecting the kneecap to the shinbone. By preventing this, you allow the tendinitis condition to improve.

In some people, a small area of tendon can spontaneously lose its blood supply. It feels the same as tendinitis, but it is technically referred to as tendinosis. This particular variation of tendinitis doesn't respond as well to anti-inflammatory medication. (Inflammation isn't a big part of the picture.) Orthopedists occasionally treat tendinosis by surgically excising the involved area.

Just about every tendon is a candidate for tendinitis. This includes the hamstrings and funny-sounding tendons like the popliteus. The initial treatment is the same in all cases: avoidance of painful activities, a trial of anti-inflammatory medication (if these are allowed to you), and physical therapy to gently stretch and soothe the painful area.

WHAT IS A NEUROMA?

Quite a simple condition, actually. There are thousands of small nerves around the knee that supply sensation to the skin. These are the nerves that let you know when something is touching your knee or if the knee is cold or hot. Some of these nerves are visible to the naked eye; others are not. By and large they are branches of the saphenous nerve, which runs along the inner thigh. When these nerves are bruised, they send pain signals to the brain. Under the microscope you can sometimes see swelling or scarring of the nerves.

However, be aware that *bruised nerves and neuromas are not revealed on an MRI.*

The diagnosis is easy to make on a physical examination: If the skin hurts when it is lightly squeezed or when a thumbnail is gently run along it, you might have a neuroma. Injecting a little local anesthetic under the skin confirms the diagnosis.

The treatment for a neuroma involves injecting a combination of an anesthetic and a special medication. Two or three injections might be required, and if this does not work, the affected tissue under the skin of the affected area might need to be surgically removed. The result of this treatment is an area of numbness—usually this is a welcome trade-off for the person who has gone so far as to require surgery.

Considering how easy it is to diagnose a neuroma, I am surprised at how often the diagnosis is missed. The issue transcends medicine: Patients with a neuroma who have been injured at work or in a car accident are routinely labeled as malingerers and gold diggers because their MRI is negative. In fact, they have a truly painful condition that can be quite stubborn.

REFLEX SYMPATHETIC DYSTROPHY (RSD)

RSD is a disorder of the nervous system that can cause severe pain. Imagine someone placing pepper under your nose. You would sneeze. With the pepper removed, the sneezing would stop. Imagine now that you would sneeze on indefinitely, even with the pepper removed. RSD is similar in that pain persists long after the inciting event ends.

As with patella malalignment, RSD is a poorly appreciated condition. The first English-language documentation of the condition dates back to the Civil War. It goes by a number of names, including causalgia, shoulder-hand syndrome (when it occurs in the arm), Sudeck's atrophy, sympathetically maintained pain, and complex-regional-pain syndrome. Specialists in this area will tell you that there are subtle differences between these conditions, but by and large they all consist of persistent, painful misfirings of pain fibers. It is unknown at this point why a small number of people develop this "reflex," but we know that just about anything can trigger the condition: a twist, a sprain, a surgical procedure of any kind, neurological disorders, cancer, etc. In its full-blown, classic incarnation, RSD presents with exquisite, burning, unrelenting pain to even the lightest touch. Pants and bed sheets are intolerable. The skin can be quite warm and then eventually very cool. It can be reddish, purplish, or mottled. The affected joint is stiff, and the affected limb can become atrophic (skinny) and dysfunctional (i.e., dystrophic).

With RSD, severe pain persists long after the injury or the surgery.

RSD is a condition of variable expression, as not every patient presents with the classic picture. In its most elemental form, RSD can simply consist of undue pain.

The best test for RSD is a "sympathetic block." This is an injection administered just to the side of the spine (usually by an anesthesiologist), and it is designed to block the sympathetic nerves to the affected area. These nerves are part of the autonomic nervous system that controls body functions that are not under voluntary control (e.g., breathing, digesting). When these nerves are blocked with Novocain or an equivalent numbing medication, the patient with RSD suddenly feels warmth in the extremity and a relief of pain. Because the cause of sympathetic misfiring is not known, multiple treatments exist, and each targets a slightly different site. These treatments include pills, injections, and physical therapy. The key to treatment, regardless of the strategy chosen, is to institute it early, as RSD addressed early on tends to respond better and more quickly. Unfortunately, because RSD often presents in subtle forms, it can escape detection for long periods of time. An even greater shame is that insurance doctors who are not attuned to this condition often delay approval for testing and treatment.

REFERRED PAIN

The body is funny in that pain in one part of the body can actually be caused by a problem far removed. Shoulder pain, for example, can come from a sick gallbladder or a pinched nerve in the neck. Likewise, pain around the knee can come from the hip, pelvis, or back. *Note:* No *knee* MRI will detect a hip or back problem. Children are particularly prone to having hip problems manifesting only as knee pain, but they can happen at any age.

> Knee pain can come from the hip or the back!

On average, I see two patients a year in need of hip-replacement surgery whose only symptoms are about the knee. More commonly, a pinched nerve in the lower back will cause radiating pain anywhere down the leg, including the knee, that may not be associated with any back pain! When the clinical and radiographic examination of the knee is perfectly normal—or not abnormal enough to account for the severity of knee symptoms—the doctor will turn his attention to other causes of knee pain, including the referred pain just described. Things become more difficult when there are enough findings about the knee to account for the knee pain. The doctor treats those findings (sometimes for quite a long time), and then, to everyone's dismay, the original symptoms persist. They do so because the knee findings were only part of the problem to begin with! Let me quickly point out that when this happens, it doesn't automatically mean that the doctor has been ignorant or negligent. However, faced with someone with persistent, unexplained knee pain, the surgeon, at some point, has to start looking elsewhere.

The following entities are not likely to be missed, but it may take a while for the diagnosis to become clear. This is especially true if the conditions do not manifest themselves in a classic manner.

OSGOOD-SCHLATTER'S

Often pronounced "osgoodschlitis" by the public, this condition was described by two doctors. (You guessed it: Osgood and Schlatter.) It consists of a painful swelling of the upper shin, and as painful as it is, it is not serious. It occurs most often in young teenagers and tends to improve on its own over time. The problem is that neither the child nor the parents are usually in the mood to simply wait it out. It is therefore worth trying a number of nonoperative measures, such as activity modification, anti-inflammatory medication, physical therapy, and knee braces. A key point here is that, in some teenagers, Osgood-Schlatter's is associated with a mild disorder of the kneecap, and *this aspect of the condition is commonly missed.* When there is such an associated disorder, it is worth reviewing it with the family. It is important for the parents to know, for example, that their child may have knee problems in the future. They may perhaps want to steer the child away from certain athletic activities. This is part of an "informed consumer" discussion. At the very least, the family will believe their child when he or she complains of pain.

RHEUMATISM

This commonly used term doesn't actually exist in the world of medicine. There are, however, a host of rheumatological conditions within the world of rheumatology. These include a large number of nontraumatic afflictions of joints and muscles, such as rheumatoid arthritis, psoriatic arthritis, lupus, Reiter's syndrome, and gout, to name but a few. These are all disorders affecting the entire body. Not every part of the body need be symptomatic, though, and the pain can start in just one area, for example, the knee. When one of these conditions is present, one or more blood tests will be abnormal. For example, when a person suffers from gout, the uric acid level is elevated, and in rheumatoid arthritis, the rheumatoid factor and sedimentation rate are elevated. Early on, nevertheless, all tests can be normal.

A few rheumatological diseases are currently known to be associated with genetic markers, and a rheumatologist is the expert with whom one should discuss these topics. Classically, rheumatological conditions (also known as "inflammatory" conditions) present with swelling, heat and redness about the knee, and occasionally a generalized fever—but not necessarily. Sometimes, the knee simply hurts.

BONE "STROKES"

Some of the more mysterious conditions about the knee involve a loss of blood flow to a part of the bone, usually the femur (thighbone). In that sense, I liken them to a stroke. In adolescents and young adults, the condition goes by the name *osteochondritis dessicans* (abbreviated OCD), and in adults it is called *osteonecrosis* or *avascular necrosis* (aka aseptic necrosis, AVN; fig. 7.2). AVN usually occurs in adults in their sixties, but it can occur both earlier and later.

OCD is treated nonoperatively in young teenagers but requires surgery in older patients when a flake of cartilage-covered bone becomes detached. The younger the patient, the better the prognosis. AVN does not involve such flaking off of bone, but a segment of bone does literally die. The segment of bone can be small, and the patient can recover quite well, or it can be large and eventually require major surgery. Most significantly, from a diagnostic point of view, the pain can come out of the blue. The person develops sudden, intense knee pain for no apparent reason. Although I have previously stated that MRIs are vastly overprescribed, the onset of sudden knee pain in someone over the age of fifty-five is a good indication for an MRI if X rays are unremarkable.

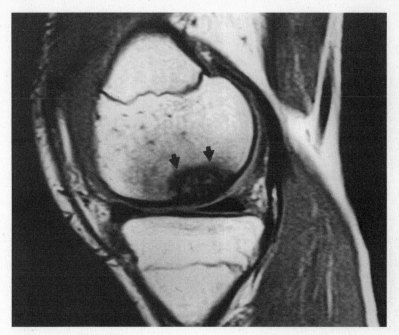

Fig. 7.2. An MRI representation of osteonecrosis (aka aseptic necrosis, avascular necrosis, *arrows*). This is akin to a stroke of the bone: An area of bone is suddenly deprived of blood supply.

LYME DISEASE

Lyme disease features a typical rash, but the rash is fleeting. Thereafter, it can manifest itself in myriad ways—knee pain being one. Lyme disease is relatively rare compared to the conditions listed above and will not be at the top of anybody's list. It may not make it at all onto an orthopedist's list. Moreover, testing for Lyme can be imperfect, and tests need to be ordered more than once if the patient is felt to be at particular risk. In certain parts of the country, doctors testing for rheumatism will automatically test for Lyme.

LIGAMENT INSTABILITY

When one or both of the cruciate ligaments are torn (see chapter 4), major instability can ensue; for example, the knee can slip in and out (the thighbone slipping over the shinbone). But in some patients the instability can be minor enough to be undetected but major enough to cause pain. This is not a common cause of pain, and the mechanism by which pain is produced remains mysterious. It is not even clear whether this diagnosis is currently over- or underdiagnosed.

BURSITIS

A bursa is a structure commonly found around joints, especially the large joints, such as the knee, hip, and shoulder. In its normal state, it is akin to a small, oily balloon, and it helps to provide smooth, painless motion about joints. When inflamed, a bursa turns into a water balloon. It swells and becomes painful. The condition is called "bursitis."

Around the knee, the bursa most likely to become inflamed is the one that lies over the kneecap. The diagnosis is easy to make because there is such obvious swelling directly over the front of the knee. The bursa can become inflamed as a result of direct trauma; for example, landing directly onto the knee. In this case, the bursa is filled with blood. The bursa can also become inflamed as a result of repeated rubbing, as can happen in someone who works on his or her knees. Here the fluid is likely to be yellow and nonbloody.

The treatment for bursitis depends in part on how much swelling is present and how much pain the patient is in. At one extreme, the condition can be observed; at the other, a needle is placed into the distended bursa and the fluid is aspirated (drawn out with a needle). Occasionally, the fluid continues to reaccumulate, and surgery is required to remove part of the bursa and to allow the tissues to scar down.

> So common in the shoulder, bursitis is relatively rare in the knee.

PIGMENTED VILLONODULAR SYNOVITIS (PVNS)/OSTEOCHONDROMATOSIS

The knee is lined with a glistening layer of tissue, in the same way that all the walls of a room might be covered with carpeting. This lining is called synovium. In normal conditions, it secretes a small amount of fluid (synovial fluid), which, among other things, provides lubrication for the joint. Tumors can grow from this synovial tissue and secrete abnormal, bloody fluid (as in PVNS) and even bits of tissue resembling grains of rice (osteochondromatosis).

These conditions are not visible on an X ray. The diagnosis is made on an MRI or is revealed at the time of an arthroscopy. These are not cancerous conditions: They do not spread to other parts of the body. They can involve just a small part of the knee or a major portion of it. They can be relatively indolent or they can be aggressive, in which case they grow quickly and destroy the tissues in their immediate vicinity. They are usually well treated by an arthroscopy (see chapter 3), but the more aggressive tumors recur.

INFECTION

Infections can occur anywhere in the body, including the knee. The typical infection causes pain, swelling, redness, and fever, which can also be the presentation of gout and other "rheumatisms" and is therefore a potential source of confusion. Infections about the knee are treated with antibiotics. The knee may also be aspirated or washed out in the operating room by means of an arthroscopy. A rare cause of infection in the knee is tuberculosis, which, in the United States, is likely to go unrecognized for a long time.

TUMORS

Tumors can exist about the knee, as they can anywhere else in the body. As with all tumors, they are divided into those that are malignant (cancerous) and those that are benign. Benign tumors cause damage in the area where they grow but by and large do not spread to other parts of the body. The list of potential tumors about the knee is remarkably long. Fortunately, if your doctor suspects a tumor, there are a number of tests available today that will provide a rapid diagnosis.

In summary, mysterious knee pain is a team approach involving the orthopedist, the rheumatologist, the neurologist, the physical therapist, and the family doctor—not necessarily in that order. If your doctor can't seem to find the cause of your pain, obtain opinions from doctors and therapists in these various fields.

Chapter 8

Does Anyone Here Know How to Take an X ray?

CONTRARY TO WHAT YOU MIGHT HAVE BEEN LED TO BELIEVE, a vast amount of information can be obtained from X rays provided that the appropriate views are obtained and the quality of the pictures is reasonable. Nevertheless, by and large, patients have poor X rays taken, and they are then immediately sent for an expensive MRI. It is true that on occasion an MRI provides critical nuggets of information that could never have been detected on X rays. More commonly, though, the MRI provides information that can be obtained from a half-decent physical examination and plain X rays. You might also be surprised to find that plain X rays can occasionally provide information not found on an MRI. Moreover, it is not uncommon with knee pain for the MRI to be frankly misleading (see chapter 2).

> A proper X ray usually obviates the need for an MRI.

Unless you are being x-rayed in an orthopedist's office, chances are that the X rays obtained will be of the so-called AP and lateral type. AP stands for anteroposterior (fig. 8.1). This means that the X-ray beam is going from front to back. A "lateral" is a side view. These two X rays represent a mug shot of your knee. They are quickly performed and are inexpensive. They are adequate for detecting major fractures and moderate-to-severe arthritis. For this reason, these are the views obtained in an emergency room. For many patients, though, these X rays are inadequate.

Arthritis, by definition, is a wearing down of the cartilage

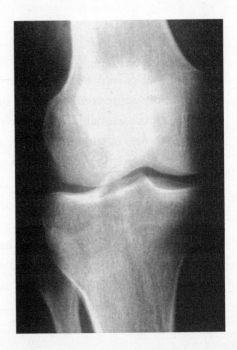

Fig. 8.1. A normal AP (front-to-back) X ray. Note the space between the femur on top and the tibia on the bottom.

lining the ends of bones. When this wearing down occurs over a large portion of the knee, the bones appear to be touching each other on an X ray, and this can be seen on the routine AP X ray described above. If, however, the wear occurs over a small area, it may be missed. If the X ray is taken with the patient in a *standing position,* however, narrowing of the space between the thighbone and the shinbone may become apparent. In such a case, the diagnosis of arthritis is made, and an MRI becomes totally superfluous.

> A satisfactory radiographic examination usually requires three X rays.

In more subtle cases, the location of the arthritis within the knee dictates that the knees be bent during the taking of the X ray. This has been called the *schuss view,* a crude reference to the position of a schussing skier (figs. 8.2 A & B). If a middle-aged patient comes to me with knee pain and I suspect subtle arthritis, I will often obtain this view. Again, if narrowing of the space between the bones is detected on this view, the diagnosis is made, and an MRI is completely unnecessary. Compared to the cost of an MRI, a schuss view is practically free.

> When arthritis is a diagnostic possibility, the "front" view has to be taken with the subject standing!

Arthritis is not the only condition that can be diagnosed by an X ray. More unusual conditions, such as osteochondritis dessicans (OCD) and avascular necrosis (see chapter 6), can also be

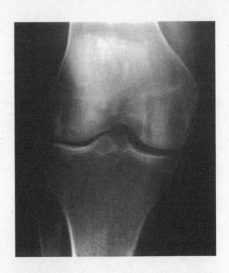

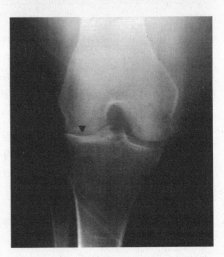

Fig. 8.2. Subtle arthritis.
A. Mild narrowing (arthritis) on a regular standing X ray (right).
B. Severe narrowing (arthritis) is apparent when this person stood with her knee bent (arrow). No MRI was necessary to diagnose her condition.

detected on an X ray. These conditions occasionally require a so-called tunnel view: The patient lies on the X-ray table, and an X ray is taken with the knee bent about 45 degrees. If you will, this is a schuss view taken with the patient lying down. (The tunnel

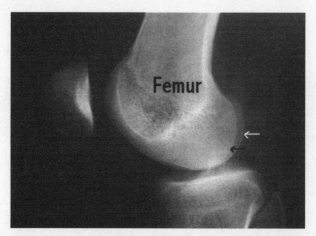

Fig. 8.3. The "true lateral" X ray. This view, which is popular in Europe, is known to only a small minority of orthopedists and radiologists in the United States. In this view the two knobs (condyles) at the end of the thighbone (femur) are superimposed (closely superimposed on this view). Each arrow represents one condyle. The X ray is striking the end of the bone at a perfect right angle. When this criterion is met, the doctor can make critical evaluations of the groove (trochlea) in which the kneecap glides. When, on the contrary, the femur is rotated relative to the X ray (which is what happens when no particular effort is made with respect to obtaining a perfect view), no information can be obtained with respect to the trochlea, and a valuable opportunity has been lost.

view is easier for the technician than the schuss view.) Bone spurs (which are always associated with arthritis) will occasionally lie in parts of the knee only visible on a tunnel view.

In patients under the age of forty-five, the *kneecap* is one of the most common sources of knee pain. If, in a given patient, the physical examination suggests that this might be the case, an X ray can help confirm the diagnosis. Again, inexpensive but appropriate views need to be obtained. These views include a

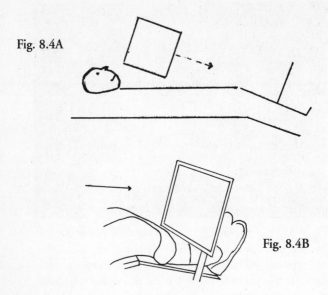

Fig. 8.4A

Fig. 8.4B

Fig. 8.4 A & B. To see whether a kneecap is out of alignment, the patient must be positioned with the legs draped over the end of the X-ray table. The X-ray beam comes from the chest and goes down to the knees. This is the "Merchant view." The cost of the special equipment is half the cost of just one MRI.

"true" lateral (fig. 8.3) and a Merchant view (figs. 8.4 A–D). A Merchant view (first described by Alan Merchant, M.D., from California) involves draping the knees over a simple device that is placed at the end of the X ray table. The device keeps the knees bent a specific number of degrees, most commonly 30 or 45 degrees. The less bent the better, for kneecap malalignment is best detected with the knee just slightly bent. Without this inexpensive device (it costs just half of one MRI test), it is impossible to make a good assessment of the kneecap's alignment. If the physical examination strongly suggests that the problem lies with the kneecap and if a kneecap abnormality is detected on the Merchant view or true lateral view, the initial diagnosis is

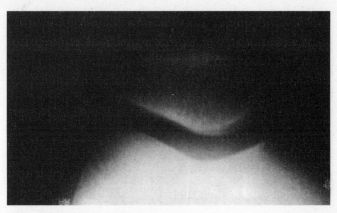

Fig. 8.4C. A normal Merchant view.

made. *No MRI is necessary at this point,* and the patient can safely be treated for the kneecap problem. Such problems usually improve with simple, nonoperative programs (see chapter 6).

Note that in some patients arthritis is localized to the kneecap, which only a Merchant view will detect. Merchant views, therefore, are also worthwhile in patients over the age of forty-five.

WHAT IS WRONG WITH SIMPLY GETTING AN MRI?

It is expensive and often does not even give you all the requisite information. Add the cost of all the unnecessary MRIs and you get a hefty figure. This affects your premiums, and it affects the insurance companies' ability to pay for other tests and treatments. Most often it is unnecessary. Conditions your doctor is looking for are often detected on appropriate X rays.

The MRI can miss conditions that an X ray will detect. In-

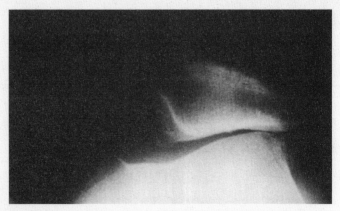

Fig. 8.4D. An abnormal view. The kneecap is tilted, it has slipped off to the right, and there is very little space left between it and the underlying thighbone (i.e., it is arthritic).

deed, the MRI is performed with the patient lying down, muscles relaxed. This is not the position in which a knee usually hurts! Subtle cases of arthritis can be completely missed on an MRI even when they are detected on the standing AP, or schuss, view. Another condition often missed on an MRI is *chondrocalcinosis*. This mouthful of a condition simply translates to "cartilage calcium," that is, calcium in the cartilage. As important as it is to have calcium in the bones, it does not belong in cartilage! When present in cartilage, microscopic knifelike calcium crystals are released into the knee. This can cause painful swelling. Although the abnormal calcium is clearly visible on X rays, it often is not apparent on an MRI.

As we've seen, the MRI can be terribly misleading. Some radiology centers routinely read a "torn meniscus (cartilage)" on every MRI. This can be done out of ignorance or malice. In any case, such a finding often focuses the attention of the patient on an irrelevant issue. An MRI in a patient whose knee is known to be arthritic adds little, if any, useful information, and it will not affect treatment. The patient will be treated nonoperatively at first regardless of what the MRI shows and will be treated surgically if the nonoperative treatment fails. This will be true regardless of the MRI findings.

IS THERE EVER A GOOD REASON FOR OBTAINING AN MRI?

Of course. The MRI is an extraordinary test. When the doctor is truly stumped, an MRI can reveal subtle and rare conditions, such as tumors. If there has been a major injury to the knee and surgery is being contemplated, the MRI can help assess the status of soft tissues, such as the cruciate ligaments. If a patient suffers from kneecap malalignment and even the Merchant view and true lateral are normal, an MRI can sometimes detect the malalignment. If a patient is found to have OCD (see chapter 7), the MRI can be of use in planning surgery. If an older patient has the early stages of osteonecrosis (a bone stroke; see chapter 7), it may be detectable only on an MRI.

If surgery is about to be performed for, say, a truly torn cartilage, an MRI can be obtained to ensure that there is no other problem in the knee. This practice of obtaining an MRI "just to make sure there is nothing else going on" is an expensive one, considering how rare it is to find something on the MRI that will change the surgeon's mind. Still, in the United States it is an acceptable use of the MRI. (In other countries it is not acceptable. This means that we are either particularly prudent or particularly spendthrift.)

In a large majority of patients with knee pain, high quality X rays obviate the need for MRI imaging.

Chapter 9

The Placebo—
A Misunderstood Treatment

THE WONDERFUL PLACEBO EFFECT

A placebo is the strangest treatment of them all. The moment a patient discovers its method of action, it stops working. A placebo is a treatment recognized as having no clear medical benefit other than the patient's satisfaction at having received a concrete form of attention.

The word *placebo* comes from the Latin "I please you." The implication is that the treatment does nothing but satisfy the patient's need for medical attention. Remarkably, though, sometimes that's all it takes to make the problem go away! Therefore, it really is a treatment. The word *placebo* is sometimes used synonymously with "doesn't work, it's just there to fool you," and that is simply not correct. Well, not completely correct. It does indeed fool you, but it can indeed work.

Here's how a placebo works: The mere fact that a person believes in a treatment somehow makes it effective. You gotta believe. Mind over matter, you might say. Naturally, the more a person believes, the better the placebo effect.

> The placebo effect: "mind over matter."

When I sat for jury duty recently, the officer who was reviewing policies and procedures to the huddled masses in front of him made the following announcement: "The water fountain has a foot pedal and a button. Ignore the pedal. It's just a placebo. It doesn't work." Everybody laughed, but that pedal was no placebo. Had the pedal truly been a placebo, one-third of prospective jurors would have felt that just pushing the pedal had quenched their thirst! The power of a placebo is nothing short of phenomenal.

Fully *one-third* of people will get pain relief from any pill. There are many ways to look at this: It's wonderful to find that an inexpensive tablet can help so many patients. On the other hand, look at the amount of money spent on medications that are no more effective than a placebo! And we haven't talked about risks yet.

> A placebo will relieve pain in 30 percent of people!

"My friend Mary takes Pain-Go-Away for her knee and she thinks it's terrific. Stopped her pain like that!" So starts many a conversation. Patients not uncommonly come to the office hoping that I will prescribe the same medication their friend has. It's not necessarily unreasonable. That Mary feels great with Pain-Go-Away only predisposes my patient that much more toward getting a placebo benefit. On the other hand, if there are medications that are more effective than Pain-Go-Away, it's unreasonable not to take the better medication.

One of the remarkable findings is that aggressive, invasive treatments, such as surgery, also have a placebo effect. This is especially true of certain operations designed to alleviate pain, and it applies particularly to the knee. In a very limited study (not involving any of my patients), patients with knee pain underwent an arthroscopy. For this procedure, small holes called portals are made at the front of the knee. Pencil-like instruments are placed into the knee through the portals, and these instruments are used to address whatever perceived problems exist in the knee. For the purposes of this study, surgeons only made the two little portals. No instruments were inserted into the knee. I think anyone would agree that making two holes in the knee has no medicinal effect (unless we're back to releasing evil humors). Yet behold! Some of the subjects reported feeling better! It is hard to know what aspect of the treatment provided the placebo effect. Being wheeled into the operating room? Getting the intravenous in the arm? The anesthesia? The surgical pain from the two incisions? The confidence in the surgeon? The relief of really being taken seriously? Or maybe it's the whole package. As surprising as this finding might be, it really isn't so astonishing if you consider again how a placebo works: The subject needs to be impressed and to believe. The more sophisticated the treatment, the more expensive the pill, the more well known the doctor, the more impressionable the patient, the greater becomes the placebo effect. What bigger treatment is there than surgery?

GREAT EXPECTATIONS

Once upon a time doctors knew nothing, yet they sounded as though they knew everything. There was a great deal of gentle deception. Not only was this socially acceptable, it was expected. Everybody suspected that doctors had very limited knowledge. It wasn't so long ago that doctors didn't know the difference between veins and arteries. In the days of Shakespeare, doctors had no clue as to why blood could be either dark red or bright red. The term *blood pressure* did not exist. As recently as 1860, Oliver Wendell Holmes is reported to have noted that if all medications "could be sunk to the bottom of the sea, it would be all the better for mankind—and all the worse for the fishes."[1] Nevertheless, the know-it-all attitude of doctors was critical to the placebo effect—the only effect that could be expected. Nowadays, doctors still don't come close to knowing everything, but they really do have a great deal of scientific, evidence-based medical information. Because of this new knowledge, patients expect a cure every time. Since there is no longer any mystery, patients want to be part of the decision-making process. They want to be informed of choices and options. Whereas failure used to be the norm, success is now so common that failure has become unacceptable. Hence, the lawsuits and the "I had no idea things could turn out so bad" frame of mind.

This brings up a tricky issue: informed consent. Patients in the United States want to be fully informed. And I agree with this completely. I certainly want to be fully informed before I agree to any procedure—or to any medication or treatment of any kind for that matter. (Don't get me started about flu shots.)

1. M. Talbot, "The Placebo Prescription," *New York Times Magazine,* January 9, 2000.

Having said that, by the time a surgeon finishes talking about all the risks and all the potential complications, he's pretty much ruined any placebo effect he might have been counting on. In fact, now you've got a scared patient. Your patient is at risk for the reverse placebo effect! The subject is so frightened by the thought of a complication that recovery is compromised. If the placebo effect exists for the better, you have to believe that it can occur for the worse.

> The concept of "informed consent" is contrary to that of a placebo. The patient is *not* supposed to know!

Given all this placebo stuff, how, then, does the surgeon explain a procedure to a patient? In reviewing legal cases, I have commonly noted that patients complain of not having been warned of a specific complication. The law is vague on this. The surgeon is supposed to inform the patient of reasonable risks, but it is up to the surgeon to decide what constitutes "reasonable." There is no official catalog of "reasonable risk." Moreover, it's not just what the surgeon tells you; it's how he tells you. He can rapidly go through the risks in a dismissive tone of voice, or he can spell each one out in exquisite detail. In the former case, the surgeon is leading the patient down a falsely rosy path, and in the latter he is sabotaging his own practice. Who wants to be operated on by a surgeon who spends so much time talking about complications? He must have a lot of complications to be dwelling on them so much! I've seen people leave their surgeon "because he's such a downer." But if there isn't enough preoperative explaining, a lawsuit can ensue. Obviously, there is a happy medium, but you can see how tricky a balancing act it is. There is a fine line between being reassuring and being dismissive. The better doctors know how to walk that line.

Making things more complex is that some patients don't want to hear about complications. They know they will probably benefit from the planned procedure and don't want to hear anything negative. In a way, this is understandable. It keeps these patients in a positive frame of mind. They recognize that they are impressionable and subconsciously don't want to be subject to the reverse placebo effect. Unfortunately, in today's climate it is impossible not to discuss potential complications. I sometimes handle this problem by speaking to the patient's relatives. At least the family, if not the patient, is an "informed consumer."

Do you know why hospitals are now paying millions of dollars to have one of their doctors anointed "team doctor" for a professional team? Placebo. Patients want to be treated by the doctor who treats their favorite athletes. If the doctor is treating well-known athletes, he has to be good, right? The patient now has just one degree of separation from their athletic hero! Their chest swells with pride at the mere thought of this association. They're psyched! Their knee *has* to get better. And the fact is, it often does. Then they refer their friends.

THE DOWN SIDE

So why do placebos get such a bad rap? Money, risks, and diversion. Let us start with diversion. Effective treatments exist for many conditions. For example, if you've just had an outpatient knee operation, we know that certain narcotics will control the pain. If, instead, someone offers you a placebo that, by definition, may or may not work, they are diverting you away from a sure thing.

> Go ahead and use a placebo when a more reliable op-
> tion doesn't exist.

This may not be serious when we are dealing "only" with
pain. After all, you can always switch back to a proven pain
medication. But it is certainly serious if you are treating an infection, a heart attack, cancer, or any other condition where
time is critical. Serious harm could befall you if you wasted pre-
cious time on a placebo.

Risks. It's one thing if a placebo is harmless; it's quite another
if there are significant risks associated with its use. The Hippo-
cratic oath taken by every medical student states "and first do no
harm." A little starch pill won't do you any harm, nor will water
with a small amount of FDA-approved coloring in it. But a pill
that can affect your kidney or a treatment associated with surgical complications is quite another story. *All* pills have potential
side effects, as, of course, does surgery. It's one thing to take a
chance on a treatment that has a very good chance of working;
it's another to take that same chance on a treatment with a
much lower success rate.

Money. Somebody's paying for your treatment. It may even
be you. In fact, it's definitely you. It's just a question of whether
you are paying directly or via premiums to an insurance company or taxes. No one minds paying for safe and effective treatments. Placebos, though, aren't predictable in their effectiveness,
nor, for knee pain, do they really work well more than 30 percent of the time. No insurance (including the government)
wants to shell out money for those kinds of odds. Too bad in a
way, because an expensive medication is going to have a better
placebo effect than an inexpensive one! Think about it: What
works better: a prescription for Naproxen, 250 milligrams twice

a day, or over-the-counter Aleve that you take twice a day? The two are essentially the same. I rest my case.

REALITY

The FDA does not give its seal of approval to pain medications that are felt to be placebos. "Why not?" you ask. "If people want to take a placebo, isn't it their own business? Is this not a free country, darn it!" Well, yes, but here's the catch: If you tell people that you are selling a placebo, its effect will be lost! One has to believe it's real medication. And if you don't tell people it's a placebo, then you're guilty of deception. The government is not into that—at least not at this level.

Manufacturers of "nutritional supplements" don't have such qualms. A nutritional supplement is a product found in nature. It hasn't been created by mankind. It is something you might ingest in common food products. These nutritional supplements generally fall outside the purview of the FDA. Manufacturers make many claims for these products. Some of them are true; some are not. Some are impossible to prove or disprove at this point. For example, if someone claims that a certain product will make us live longer, who's going to know if that's true or not until we're all gone? Some supplements work because of a specific scientific principle; others work purely on a placebo effect; in still other cases it isn't clear at all. Glucosamine and chondroitin sulfate fall into this latter category (see chapter 5). In any case, people buy nutritional supplements in huge quantities, out of their own pocket (no insurance pays for this), and if they feel better from the placebo effect, so be it. I must say, however, that I've always been somewhat surprised at how people will spend large sums of money on supplements (most of which are expensive) but then squawk when they have to fork over the ten-dollar copay for their office visit.

REAL MEDICINE VERSUS PLACEBOS

How does the FDA protect us from placebos? It demands "controlled clinical trials." One group of patients gets the new medication, and another group gets a pill that looks the same but is made of a (presumably) inert substance. Ideally, the study is "double blind": Neither the doctor nor the patient knows whether he or she is getting the medication or the placebo. They just know it as A or B. After a period of time, the code is revealed. Everyone then knows who got what, and the effectiveness of the medication can be compared to that of the placebo. In fact, that's how people discovered that placebos work! Because even in the placebo group people got better!

In order for a medication to be approved by the FDA, it has to be deemed safe (though no medication is 100 percent safe), and it has to work better than a placebo. Is a 30 percent success rate good enough for the FDA? If a placebo works on 2 percent of subjects, the answer is yes. If, however, a placebo was found to work on 29 percent of patients tested, the answer is no! When it comes to pain, that's the success rate that we're talking about. So if 30 percent of your friends who've tried this new, "natural" pain medication tell you they love it, they're just getting a placebo effect. But don't tell them; you'll ruin it for them. Placebos *über alles?*

It is not terribly surprising to find that a placebo alleviates pain. Pain is not a monolithic entity. It's more like a layered cake. There's the actual pain, and there is the anxiety associated with it. In some cases, the anxiety component is by far the major factor, and it's easy to see how the power of suggestion could address this.

I find this all the time when giving injections. Some people clench their fists, break out into a sweat, and cry for their mother at the mere mention of an injection, while others coolly file their nails.

It is harder to imagine how a placebo affects conditions seemingly unrelated to anxiety. The chest pain you get from shoveling snow is due to a lack of oxygen to your heart and is called angina. Parkinson's is a degenerative condition of certain brain cells that can lead to stiffness and tremors. Colitis is an inflammation of the colon. Asthma is a constriction of the air ducts in the lungs. Warts are nasty growths. None of these conditions should be amenable to a placebo, yet all have been found to be. Where does it end?

Unfortunately, people still get sick and die even when they fervently believe. Cancer is an area that has not been vanquished by placebos. It is therefore a dangerous area in which to fool around. The same holds true for bacterial infections. People used to die from what today would be called simple infections. Appendicitis was a killer. (Even Houdini could not escape.) If you develop a bacterial infection, you want an evidence-based medication

A LITTLE RESPECT

What, then, should be organized medicine's stand on placebos? Once upon a time, placebos, these "lies that heal," were just about the only form of treatment available. Though they could not cure cancer or arrows through the heart, they helped a large number of patients afflicted with a remarkable array of conditions.

> Once upon a time placebos were the only treatments available to doctors and patients.

No one questioned the doctor about his treatment. He was above reproach. Everyone knew that the doctor's cure rate was limited, but any chance of success lay greatly in belief.

Society has now turned 180 degrees. We expect victory and want no part of any phony-baloney. The doctor has been stripped of mystery and magic. Instead of the haughty, paternalistic physician who looks down his nose through those little glasses and tells you you'll get better, you have the kinder, gentler doctor who tells you about all the terrible things than can go wrong. We are winning the battle over conditions that require science and losing out on those that just need a little placebo. Doctors no longer dare be paternalistic. Society does not accept this.

If a treatment is no better than a placebo, it is reasonable to abandon the treatment, especially if it is expensive or risky. But how about the placebo itself? If, by definition, it is harmless, why not adopt it as a treatment if it can help some patients?

We have arrived at an interesting point in our medical advances: We understand that diseases all have a scientific basis, and we have developed scientific treatments for many of these conditions. *Many,* not all. And yet for the conditions that we do not fully understand and for which we do not have fully safe and effective treatments, we refuse to allow placebos into our armementarium. We know enough to understand that all treatments should be scientific, that is, evidence-based, but we don't have enough knowledge to implement this safely and effectively across the board. Until then, maybe we should take a more scientific look at placebos.

Chapter 10

Injuring Your Knee in the Name of Health

CHANCES ARE THAT YOU EXERCISE. YOU DO SO BECAUSE IT'S fun, or you want to keep your weight down, or it's a way to stay in touch with people, or because everyone else is, or your doctor told you to, or you feel it will keep you healthy.

These are all good reasons to exercise. However, not all forms of exercise are good for your knee. And it is one thing to injure your knee while having fun; it's quite another thing to hurt it while going through some tedious routine because it is good for you!

Generally speaking, there are two ways you can hurt your knee: by way of a sudden event or via repetitive use. The former is easy to understand: If you stress the bones, ligaments, tendons, or cartilage beyond a certain point, they will fail. The repetitive injury is more subtle. You can't trace the pain back to any one single event. You're not even sure that your athletic activity triggered the symptoms, but your sport aggravates the pain. Some repetitive injuries are the result of overuse, that is, you've simply done more than what your body can tolerate. You can occasionally overcome this through training, but at other times you've simply pushed your envelope as far as it will go. Other repetitive injuries are the result of faulty techniques or equipment, and these should be easier to address. Let us look at some athletic activities:

RUNNING

Running (or jogging) has arguably been the sport most affected by the fitness ardor of the last twenty years. Initially, there was concern among sports-medicine doctors that pounding on the knee, mile after mile, would lead to early *arthritis* among running enthusiasts. This fear has not materialized. A healthy, well-aligned knee appears to tolerate running quite well. Of course, we do not yet know the thirty- and forty-year effects of repeated, prolonged running, but early results are encouraging.

And yet some vigilance is warranted. Note that I stated that "a well-aligned knee" appears to tolerate running. People who are bowlegged or knock-kneed are at risk for arthritis in the first place (see chapter 7) because they tend to place all their weight on just one part of the knee. Although there is, as yet, no conclusive proof of this, it stands to reason that such people may be at even greater risk of arthritis with years of repetitive jogging. I do not recommend jogging to my bowlegged and knock-kneed patients.

As the knee bends and straightens, a thick band of tissue running along the outside of the thigh rubs back and forth along the side of the femur (thighbone). This band is called the iliotibial

(ITB) band because it starts high up on the ilium bone (one of the pelvic bones) and runs along the thigh all the way down to the tibia (shinbone). In some people, the repetitive rubbing eventually leads to inflammation and pain (see chapter 7). Because the pain is localized in the outside part of the knee joint, the unwary practitioner may suggest that you have torn cartilage. As we have stated a few times already in this book, this misdiagnosis is even more likely if you have had the misfortune of undergoing an MRI. In the old days, if a patient said, "It hurts when I do this," the doctor's obvious retort was "Well, don't do this!" That is no longer acceptable. A sports-medicine doctor's goal is to get his or her patients back to the activities they love. Nevertheless, part of your treatment will involve cutting back temporarily on your mileage. Stretching, cold packs, anti-inflammatory medications, perhaps physical therapy and injections, will be included in the treatment package, after which you can gradually begin to increase your mileage (see chapter 11).

You should evaluate your *running routine*. Are you increasing your mileage too rapidly? A 10 percent increase per week has been regarded as a maximum, but for you even this might be too much. Everybody is different. Listen to your body rather than blindly obeying a formula. Are you running on concrete? Of course, you may not have much choice, but rock-hard surfaces are obviously going to be tougher on your knees. Are you running on hills? Hills are problematic whether you are running up, down, or sideways. Running up or down places stress on your kneecap, and it puts you at risk for developing pain in the patellofemoral (kneecap) joint. Running sideways on a hill puts your feet and legs at an unnatural angle, and it predisposes you to having pain anywhere from your back down to your feet.

The shoes one wears are critical. The running shoe is designed to absorb shock as the foot strikes the ground. It is also designed to support the delicate and intricate mechanism of foot mechanics—the complex interaction of the many bones and ligaments inside the foot during weight-bearing activities. Without a good shoe, the ligaments in the foot would begin to stretch painfully after prolonged running, and the repeated pounding would cause added inflammation. Therefore, a cardinal rule is to ensure that your shoes are in good condition.

Are you flat-footed? You look under your foot, you see an arch, and you say no. Sorry, that's not how to tell. Unless you are severely flat-footed, the arch looks fine until you stand and put all your weight on the foot. Normally, the arch does not touch the ground. (Check out footprints in the sand.) If you are flat-footed, it will. An approximate synonym for being flat-footed is "foot pronation," as in "the foot pronates abnormally." Many scientific (and pseudoscientific) articles have been devoted to the effect of abnormal foot mechanics on knee pain. Although controversy still exists as to just how altered foot mechanics can cause knee pain, there is no question that the correlation exists. If your feet are flat when you run, you are at increased risk of developing knee pain. Presumably, your foot twists as it strikes the ground, and this twist gets transmitted up the leg, which then generates abnormal, painful stresses about the knee. That is as specific as I can get without wading into unsubstantiated theories.

Most running shoes have a built-in arch support, which is in contradistinction to the traditional "sneakers," where the insole is completely flat. Therefore, for most runners, a regular running shoe will suffice. Even an arch that is slightly flat will be adequately supported by the insole of a running shoe. If, however, your foot is very flat, the insole of your running shoe will not do. You may need an orthotic, an insert that is slipped into your shoe. Such a device will support the arch, restore more normal foot mechanics, and, one hopes, minimize knee pain.

Though flat feet represent the most common foot abnormality, there are many other variations of foot anatomy. They can all potentially predispose to pain. If your foot looks funny in any way and your knee hurts when you run, consider obtaining an orthopedic or a podiatric consultation. You may benefit from an orthotic in your running shoe.

AT THE GYM

"I go to the gym" is the answer most people give when I ask whether they exercise. Of all the athletic activities available out there, gym exercises are the ones most likely to be performed strictly for health. Going to the gym represents a commitment to stay or become fit. Although clearly there can be a social aspect to doing so, few people go to the gym for fun. It is therefore particularly vexing to get injured at the gym, for this is the ultimate example of injuring yourself in the name of health.

Sudden injuries are incurred when the knee is simultaneously (and rapidly) bent and twisted, as when going from a jump to a squat while turning the torso. The meniscus can pop (see chapter 3) and require surgery. The same can happen if you get up suddenly from an awkward position. If you suffer from kneecap malalignment (see chapter 6), the kneecap can slip out of its groove when you plant your foot and twist your upper body. Turning (with the feet planted on the ground) to throw a basketball is an example of such an activity. You should avoid it if you've ever been told that your kneecap "went out" or that your "patella subluxated" or that your "patella dislocated." If you're into lifting weights, you can rupture the patellar tendon while "jerking" weights that are too heavy for you. This injury will also require surgery and will be associated with a lengthy rehabilitation period. Lunging activities can cause a "pulled" muscle in the calf or thigh—an actual tear of muscle fibers. It is associated with sudden pain, swelling, and discoloration of the skin over a period of a few days. To a certain extent, stretching prior to exercising can prevent muscle pulls. To obtain maximum benefit from stretching, the stretch must be maintained for twenty seconds!

Most knee injuries at the gym are related to overuse, that is, excessive repetition of flexion/extension (bending/straightening). *Overuse* is the medical term for overdoing it. As can happen with running, a knee that is repeatedly bent and straightened is prone to developing tendinitis. If you go through a stair or step routine, you may develop pain in your kneecap. Such injuries are relatively easy to treat to the extent that they require simple analgesics, anti-inflammatory medications, ice, and activity modification.

RACKET SPORTS

All racket sports involve considerable bending and twisting from the torso on down. Although tennis elbow, by virtue of its appellation, would seem to be the most common tennis injury, knee pain can't be far behind. Once again, overuse is the major culprit. The "weekend warrior" syndrome brings people into the office Monday mornings. Players are sore from having simply overdone it. The pain can be anywhere about the knee, and the error here is for the doctor to send the tennis player for an MRI, unless one or the other is looking for surgery. Barring a sudden injury, the problem is not likely to be a meniscus despite the inevitable "torn cartilage" on the MRI report.

Sudden knee injuries are rare in racket sports, although an awkward twist can certainly pop a meniscus or strain a ligament. Moreover, planting the foot and turning the body is de rigueur in these sports, and the kneecap can slip out of its groove in people with a predisposition to this problem. The best way to prevent such injuries is to play on surfaces with some give, such as clay. By allowing the foot to swivel, torque at the knee level is minimized. Common, over-the-counter braces, on the other hand, are not likely to prevent an injury. Nevertheless, some players feel more secure with an elastic support around the knee, in which case I give my blessing to its use.

BASKETBALL

Anyone who plays basketball probably follows the sport enough to read the sports pages. And anyone reading the sports pages knows how often basketball players injure their knees. Although ankle sprains are probably more common, knee injuries tend to be more serious.

That serious knee injuries should occur commonly in this sport is hardly a surprise. Lunging, jumping, and landing awkwardly are part and parcel of the game. The accidents incurred span the entire gamut of available injuries: medial collateral ligament (MCL) sprains, anterior cruciate ligament (ACL) and posterior cruciate ligament (PCL) tears, meniscal tears, and kneecap dislocations. Not to mention combinations of the above. The "terrible triad" is a particularly pernicious combination of an MCL, ACL, and medial meniscal tear.

As any college or professional player will tell you, there is no way to completely prevent these injuries, though it never hurts to be in shape. The more you weigh, the more torque is applied to your knee when you land from a jump.

Women are far more likely than their male counterparts to sustain ACL tears (see chapter 4). Though the reasons for this are still subject to debate, the fact that a major discrepancy exists between the sexes is not.

According to one of the more prevalent theories, women tend to land from a jump in a more stiff-legged manner, which is quite an optimistic hypothesis, because the problem should be amenable to training. And the very preliminary results are encouraging: Centers that have focused on jumping and landing skills have noted a decrease in women's ligament injuries. This is still a very young field, however, and many questions remain unanswered.

"Jumper's knee" is specific to basketball. Pain develops toward the front of the knee as a result of repeated jumping. The pain is caused by an inflammation of the patellar tendon, which connects the kneecap to the shinbone (tibia). Though less worrisome than the injuries listed above, it can, nonetheless, be a stubborn condition. The treatment is standard fare for tendon inflammations: rest, ice, and anti-inflammatory medications. On rare occasion, chronically abnormal tissue forms within the tendon, which can require surgery.

SOCCER

With respect to the knee, soccer is similar to basketball. One leg has to be planted while the other kicks, and on the side that is planted, the knee is subject to major twisting forces. Moreover, players are constantly sliding into each other, and this adds another dimension of risk. Thus, all the injuries described for basketball are also common in soccer.

Once again, women are even more at risk. Stretching, conditioning, and keeping one's weight down all improve the odds against serious injury, but soccer remains a high-risk activity with respect to the knee.

GOLF

How harmful to the knees can golf be? It involves no running or jumping. And yet stress on the knees associated with lugging a dead weight around for a few miles is obvious if you consider golf a sport and carry or pull your clubs around the course. As far as your knees are concerned, you just gained an awful amount of weight. It is obviously milder on the knees if you consider golf more a skill than a sport and you navigate the course in a golf cart. But the golf swing still involves twisting. Depending on the exact nature of your knee condition, it may or may not present a problem. For example, if you have a torn meniscus (torn cartilage), the twisting motion of the knee may tug on the tear, which can be painful. The tear only has to be a fraction of an inch removed for this same motion to be painless. The same holds for arthritis. If it's in just the wrong spot, the pain of wear and tear can be exacerbated by a golf swing. In both the cases of a torn cartilage and arthritis, you are not harming yourself by playing golf—just causing more pain. You might take some pain medication just before playing (e.g., a combination of an anti-inflammatory medication if your doctor allows it and some acetaminophen).

If your kneecap tends to slip in and out (see chapter 6), the golf swing can put your kneecap at risk. You would have discovered this early in your golf career. In this situation, bracing of the knee can be helpful. (You need a so-called patellofemoral knee support.)

SKIING

Contrary to basketball and soccer, ski injuries can be minimized by training and proper maintenance of equipment. In the typical ski injury, the tip of the ski gets caught. The ski veers off to the side, while the other ski continues to point straight ahead. "Pop" goes the medial collateral ligament (MCL) of the knee that's veering off. The better the skier, the less likely this injury is to occur. The anterior cruciate ligament (ACL) is also at risk during skiing. According to a University of Vermont study, among recreational skiers this injury is most likely to occur when the skier allows him or herself to fall back in a sitting, "hip below knee" position. If one ski diverges away from the other, the conditions are right for an ACL tear. Again, the more advanced the skier, the less likely this is to happen.

Slow, twisting injuries of the kind sustained in heavy, springlike snow can also wreak havoc on a knee, as bindings are less likely to release in these conditions.

Fortunately, ski equipment continues to improve. Bindings are becoming more sophisticated, and they release under a greater variety of conditions than in the past. Given a choice, spend the extra money on bindings rather than on skis. On a more negative note, ski boots are higher and more rigid than those of twenty years ago, and torque has been transmitted higher up the leg: "Boot top" fractures of the shinbone (tibia) have given way to ligament injuries about the knee. Moreover, bindings that are not regularly cleaned and lubricated will tend to jam, thus nullifying any improvement in technology.

Collisions between skiers remain a danger against which expertise and equipment are powerless. Collisions are a particular problem in resorts that do not monitor overcrowding and take no steps to control speeding. These high-speed crashes lead to knee injuries more commonly seen in motor-vehicle accidents, such as multifragment fractures.

SNOWBOARDING

With both feet attached to one large board, the snowboarder does not have to worry about one leg veering off in a crazy direction. He or she is therefore relatively immune to the MCL sprain and to the ACL tear. Snowboarders are more at risk for arm injuries, having no poles to compensate for a loss of balance.

CYCLING

Among sports, bicycle riding is the leading cause of life-threatening injuries. It is not, however, a leader among isolated, serious knee trauma. Nevertheless, because repetitive bending and straightening of the knee are inherent in the sport, overuse syndromes, such as iliotibial (ITB) tendinitis, are common. Moreover, the knee can be excessively stressed if a foot that naturally turns in or out is forced by the toe clips to point forward.

WRESTLING

The wrestler can injure his medial collateral ligament (MCL), anterior cruciate ligament (ACL), or meniscus, as can any athlete who awkwardly twists his knee. In addition, the wrestler commonly lands directly on his knee, and such trauma can lead to bursitis. If the swelling and pain are mild, no specific treatment is required. On the other hand, severe pain and swelling mandate an "aspiration": placement of a needle into the swollen bursa and removing the fluid.

Chapter 11

Exercises for a Healthy Knee

TREATMENT PROTOCOLS FOR JUST ABOUT ANY KNEE CONDItion should incorporate knee exercises. The correct knee exercises. This is true whether you are trying to treat a certain condition or trying to prevent it.

Knee exercises can be part of a head-to-toe, stay-in-shape training program, or they can be the sole focus of an exercise session. Either way, they should make you feel good. They are not designed to be a form of torture. Ideally, they should be fun.

So turn on the TV, put on some dance music, and start working those knees!

An exercise program can be divided into categories:

- the aerobic warm-up
- stretching
- strengthening
- conditioning
- water exercises

STEP 1: LIGHT AEROBICS, STRETCHING OF THE SHOULDERS AND THE BACK (YES, EVEN FOR KNEE CONDITIONS)

Start the juices flowing with some basic calisthenics. This gets your body and soul into an exercise frame of mind. Run lightly in place. Hold a three- to five-pound weight in each hand. Slowly raise your arms as high as you can. (Reach for the sky.) As you strain to reach up, you should feel those tissues about the shoulders stretching, stretching, stretching.

Now, as you lower your arms, bring your shoulders way back, military style. Keep running in place. Put the weights down. Grab the back of each shoulder with the opposite hand. Inch your fingers farther and farther back. Without turning your feet, turn your torso all the way to the right and then all the way to the left. Repeat. After five minutes of this, you are ready to address the knee.

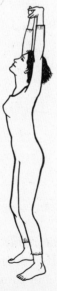

Fig. 11.1. "Reach for the sky."

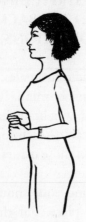

Fig. 11.2. Stand straight with your shoulders back.

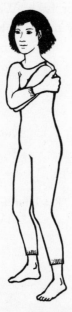

Fig. 11.3. Grab the back of your shoulders.

Note: You should be able to comfortably carry on a conversation while running. If not, stop. If your knee hurts, perform the shoulder and back stretches without running.

A basic exercise principle is "warm up, ice down." That is, if it's cold and you feel particularly stiff, warm up. Literally. If the air temperature is cool, wear warm clothing. Discard layers as you work up a light sweat. Consider applying heat directly to a stiff area by way of a warm gel pack. When you are done exercising, ice down the areas that you know will be sore. Cold reduces swelling and acts as a painkiller without side effects. If you are using ice, do not apply it directly onto the skin, but rather on a thin towel or cloth. Otherwise, you can get frostbite.

Aerobic tips

- If the temperature is cool, start by wearing a sweatsuit. As you work up a light sweat, discard the suit.
- Shoes should be light and supple. (Shoes designed for basketball are made to resist high levels of torque. Such support is not necessary here, though it is not harmful.)
- When possible, exercise in a cool, well-ventilated area. There is no benefit to profuse perspiration.

STEP 2: STRETCHING

Stretching is a key component of *any* knee program. I know, it's boring. But yes, it's *that* important. Stiffness of any muscle group hampers the normal, free-flowing motion of the knee. This slight alteration of muscle tone, sometimes invisible to the naked eye, adds pressure to parts of the knee and can exacerbate existing pain.

And it's not just the muscles that need stretching. The tendons (connecting muscles to bones) also need to get into the act. From a distance they look like ropes. Under a powerful microscope, however, one notes that they consist of millions of little biological springs. With sustained stretching, these miniature springlets uncoil somewhat, and the tendons become a little more elastic. Instead of looking like ropes, they start to behave like rubber bands. Okay, it's a slight exaggeration, but you get the point. The operative word here is "sustained." Bouncing around doesn't stretch anything. When you perform a stretching exercise, you must hold that position for twenty seconds. Those little coils don't just unwind at the snap of a finger.

Anatomically, the muscles that control the knee start high up on the leg in the area of the hip and pelvis. For example, the hamstrings at the back of the thigh originate on the so-called ischial tuberosity, the bone you sit on! One of the muscles that extend your knee (the rectus femoris) starts at the front of your abdomen, just below the belt line. At the other end of the leg, the calf muscles that raise your heels off the ground also bend the knee. In short, one way or the other, just about every muscle in the leg affects your knee. Stretching exercises for the knee therefore involve the whole leg.

Following an injury or surgery, your knee will not want to straighten all the way. And it will not want to bend. Indeed, bending or straightening stretches the ligaments and tendons, which is painful. If you give in to the knee's reluctance to straighten and bend, two things may happen: Your knee pain may persist or worsen. Moreover, you might permanently lose knee motion. "Move it or lose it," as they say in physical-therapy circles.

Home Exercises

A therapist can't be with you all day long, so you need to exercise on your own, too. Figs. 11.4–8 cover basic stretches. Note that with age, the adductors (fig. 11.7) become tight (that's why you have more trouble reaching for that tennis ball), and they need to be included in your stretching program.

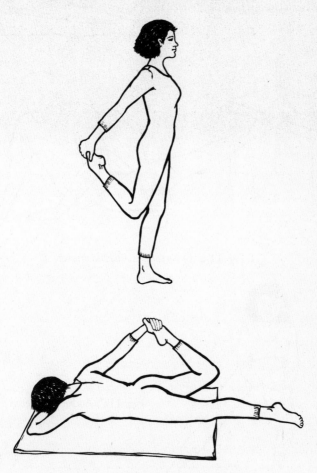

Fig. 11.4 A & B. Quadriceps stretch.

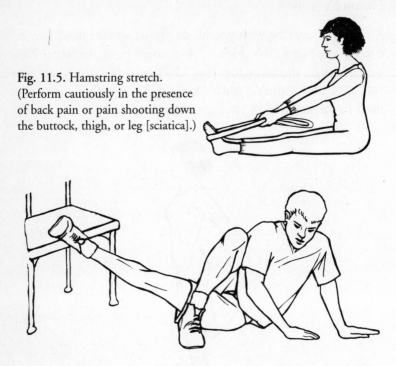

Fig. 11.5. Hamstring stretch. (Perform cautiously in the presence of back pain or pain shooting down the buttock, thigh, or leg [sciatica].)

Fig. 11.6. ITB (iliotibial band) stretch.

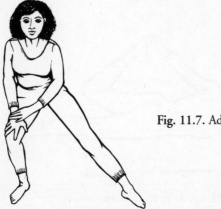

Fig. 11.7. Adductor stretch.

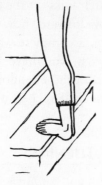

Fig. 11.8. "Gastroc" (gastrocnemius-soleus) stretch.

Trick of the trade: If you have trouble straightening the knee after surgery or after an injury, try this trick (fig. 11.9): Lie on your bed, facedown. Wiggle down to the end of the bed until the knee rests right at the edge of the bed. Then just let your leg hang down. The weight of your leg will gradually straighten out the knee. If that doesn't work well enough, put a book or two in a handbag and let the handbag hang from your ankle. Progressively add books until you feel a difference. By the way, this book has been scientifically designed to be the ideal weight. It's even more effective when you use four at once, so I advise you to rush out and buy three more copies (and tell your friends).

Keep in mind that at no point should you experience pain. As with all stretching, give the exercise time. You have to be patient.

Stretching Tips

- Stretches need to be held for twenty seconds.
- Do not bounce around from one stretching exercise to another.

How to (and not to) stretch. Watch folks on the tennis court. They lean right, they lean left, now forward, now backward, a little twist here, a little twist there, a complete waste of time. *Hold that stretch.* With each stretch, you have to count to twenty. Think of the tiny springlets in those tendons. It takes a s-u-s-t-a-i-n-e-d effort to stretch the little suckers out.

STEP 3: STRENGTHENING

Weak muscles contribute to wobbly, painful knees. To a certain extent, then, strengthening exercises can alleviate pain. But be careful! Certain exercises can themselves be painful. Such exercises are to be avoided! It is *not* a "no pain, no gain" situation.

Strengthening exercises are divided into maintenance exercises and activity-specific exercises. Maintenance exercises provide general fitness. Activity-specific exercises are geared toward training for a specific endeavor.

If you're going to strengthen your knee, you need to work on all the muscle groups discussed above (quadriceps, hamstrings, etc.).

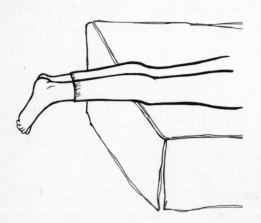

Fig. 11.9. Trick of the trade: a special *straightening* exercise following knee surgery.

Strengthening Tips

- Not "no pain, no gain"
- Start with light weights and work your way up.
- Wall slides are very tough on kneecaps. Avoid them!

The four quadriceps muscles are at the front of the thigh. They straighten the knee when it is bent, as when, for example, you want to kick a ball. When you stand and your knees are slightly bent (which is most of the time), the quads are the muscles that keep your knee from bending all the way and prevent the leg from collapsing.

To *strengthen your quadriceps,* try this exercise: Wrap a two- or three-pound ankle weight to your lower leg and sit on a chair. Straighten the knee slowly and then let your foot down (fig. 11.10). Repeat a total of ten times. Wait a few moments and repeat. Boring? You bet. Listen to some music or watch a movie. If this exercise is too easy, increase the weight. What, you don't have ankle weights? Time to pull out that handbag again. *Cau-*

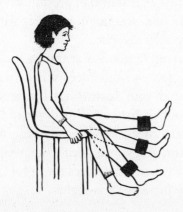

Fig. 11.10. Leg extension. Use only light weights.

tion: Increase weights very gradually. The length of your leg magnifies the effect of the weights at the level of your knee. (Remember levers in high school?) An increase of just one pound can translate to quite a bit more force on the knee.

This exercise is called a *leg extension.* As long as it does not hurt, it is safe, and it is easy to do. You can certainly do this on your own at home.

Steps—either up or down—are another way to strengthen the quads. Step exercises are a little less practical if you live in a ranch-style house or in an apartment, but in medical lingo they are more "physiological" than leg-extension exercises. This means that they approximate everyday activities more closely.

There are pitfalls with every exercise, and step exercises are no exception: The steps should not be too big. The stairs in your house or your apartment building are probably fine, but in some gyms and exercise classes you will only find large step stools. Those might be okay for you, but make sure you can handle normal steps (stairs) first.

Be careful with *wall slides!* To perform a wall slide, you stand with your back to a wall, your heels a foot or so away from the wall. You gradually slide down and get back up. The farther your feet are from the wall, the tougher the exercise. It does strengthen the quads, but it puts a great deal of pressure on your kneecaps. If your kneecaps are fine, you might get away with it, but I don't think it's a very healthy exercise.

The hamstrings consist of three muscles at the back of the thigh. They serve principally to bend the knee. When you are standing, you don't really need your hamstrings for bending purposes because gravity does this for you. But if you're lying down and want to bend your knees, you'll want those hamstrings. To strengthen the hamstrings, you need ankle weights. Lie on your stomach and slowly bend the knees (fig. 11.11). As with leg extensions, gradually increase the weights.

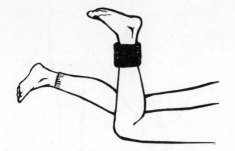

Fig. 11.11.
Hamstring
strengthening.

Perhaps you're thinking that you don't need your knees that much when you're lying down, so the heck with the hamstring exercises. (Buzzer) Wrong! Muscle actions about the knee are more complicated than simple bending and straightening. They all work in concert during every activity. More on that below.

The abductors are the muscles on the outer aspect of your thighs. Guess what they do. Yes, they abduct the leg! Translation: They swing the leg away from the body. When you are standing, the abductors raise the leg off to the side. A (male) dog abducts his leg at the fire hydrant. You can strengthen these muscles by standing with ankle weights on, abducting your leg slowly, and letting it back down. Another exciting exercise. (There's a reason for all that music in exercise classes.)

> Elastic bands can replace free weights.
> They come in different colors and stiffness.

The adductors live on the inner aspect of your thigh and have the opposite function. They bring the leg in line with your body. That happens naturally when you're standing, but if you're lying down with your leg out (say, you're doing an abduction exercise), it's the adductors that bring the leg back in. Strengthen-

Fig. 11.12. Abductor strengthening.

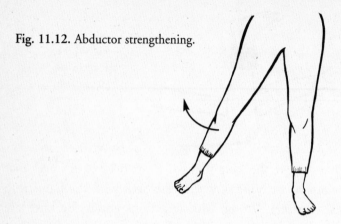

Fig. 11.13. Adductor strengthening.

ing the adductors is a little more involved because by and large gravity does their work. As soon as you lift your leg (abduct) to the side, gravity will work against the abductor muscles to bring the leg back down. Stand with a heavy concrete block between your feet (surely you have one in a closet somewhere) and try to push the block toward the other foot. Push for ten seconds and relax. Repeat until bored. That's likely to be about five seconds. So actually give yourself a target of ten repetitions and move on to another exercise (e.g., strengthening the abductors of the other leg!). If you're one of the few without a concrete block around the house, try the more ubiquitous guitar amplifier. An encyclopedia works too (less well if you have it on CD). You get the point.

Alternatively, wide *elastic bands* are commercially available. They come in different colors, each representing a certain stiffness (e.g., Theraband). You tie one end of the band around your ankle and the other end around the foot of a table. Pull your foot away from the table and you're working your adductors. If you've gone ahead and bought these bands, you might as well use them for other exercises. Sit on a chair facing a table with one end of the band around your leg and the other around a foot of the table. Pull your leg away from the table until there is no longer any slack in the band. Now bend the knee. The elastic band will offer resistance, and you will be working your hamstrings. Now, instead of tying one end of the band around a table, tie it around the foot of your chair. When you straighten your knee, the elastic band will once again offer resistance, and you will be working your quads.

STEP 4: CONDITIONING

Conditioning is the practice of getting ready for a particular activity. This is the fun part. Thank God, because as important as stretching and strengthening are, that stuff can be pretty boring.

There are two aspects of conditioning: (1) building up endurance, and (2) preparing the muscle groups to work with each other.

The concept of endurance is easy to understand. Anyone who has huffed and puffed running for a bus already knows all about it. Your heart, your lungs, your muscles, and every other fiber in your body have to gear up for prolonged activity. You accomplish this by, well, doing it. You start with a short period of exercise and build up by doing a little more with each exercise session. The common wisdom is that you should be able to carry on a conversation while exercising. If you're so out of breath that you can't talk, stop.

> If you can no longer carry on a conversation, *stop* the exercise!

The concept of preparing muscle groups to work together is less intuitive. Think of superstrong men with powerful weapons. As strong as they may be, collectively they would not make a great army their first day on the job. They have to learn to work as a team. They must anticipate the job that needs to be done and move in a coordinated manner to achieve their objectives. The same goes for your knee. Whether you're picking a quarter off the floor, climbing steps, or kicking the winning field goal, *all* muscles about your knee come into play. Naturally, if you're kicking a ball, the quads may work harder than the hamstrings, but the fact is that even the hamstrings contract. That smooth motion you get when engaging in any activity comes from the seamless interaction of the multiple muscle groups about the knee. That comes with practice.

Feedforward

You've heard of feedback. It's a response to something or someone. Feedforward is anticipation. As the ball heads your way, your muscles already know what they're going to do. Like a well-trained army, each unit knows its job. The quads will contract just so much and will do so a split second before such-and-such muscles and a split second after others. A moment later they'll relax a bit while the hamstrings kick in. Then you miss your shot, curse, and start again.

> The best way to train for an activity is to mimic it.

Show a pianist the sheet music to Für Elise, and the millions of muscle spindles in her forearm will quickly take their proper place, ready to fire at precisely the right moment. This kind of anticipation only comes with practice. Practicing Für Elise, that is! Practice Mozart's Turkish Rondo instead and your Für Elise will sound like Fürgetaboutit. In short, the only way to train for an activity is to mimic it.

STEP 5: WATER EXERCISES

The mere act of standing causes pressure on your knees. When you stand in water, chest-deep, you are suddenly much lighter. You are said to be more buoyant. (I sense that you are not surprised.) Exercises that would be too painful on land suddenly become conceivable in water.

What, you don't swim? You don't like to get your head wet? No matter. You can get plenty of exercise in the shallow end of the pool. For starters, have you ever tried running in the shallow end of the pool? It's very tiring. It's a "good" tiring, too. It's aerobic, meaning that blood is rapidly flowing through the muscles, bearing oxygen and other goodies. It doesn't raise your blood pressure because you're never straining that hard.

You can lunge forward, leap right and left, and even perform jumping jacks. The water resists your every movement and strengthens each muscle group.

Provided the water is warm enough, the pool has a limbering effect. Some of those stretches become a little easier (not the ones where you sit on the ground; avoid doing those in the pool).

This brings us to the point of pool temperature: If the water is too cold, it may actually lead you to stiffen up. So check the temperature before signing up.

Some physical-therapy outfits feature underwater treadmills. I give them a thumbs up.

The deep end of the pool opens up another array of exercises, with or without getting your head wet. A number of arm and leg attachments have been developed to increase the water's resistance as you move about. They are effective as long as you are not overworked. As noted above, in order to ensure that you are not overstressing your heart, you should be able to carry on a simple conversation while you exercise. (Instructors hate to break up a class to pull someone out of the bottom of the pool.) These resistive devices make your muscles work harder, and the muscles therefore become stronger.

When planning a vacation, it's not a bad idea to look for places that have a warm pool.

Chapter 12

Your Insurance Company and Your Knee

YOUR INSURANCE COMPANY FALLS INTO ONE OF TWO CATE-gories: Either it allows your doctor to do what he or she sees fit, or it attempts to exert some control over what your doctor recommends. Clearly, this is not just true for knee problems.

Overall, as a doctor, I find it odious that an impersonal institution that has never met my patient would try to dictate the care I prescribe. This is particularly galling when the people making these decisions (both nurses and doctors) have less expertise than I do.

On the other hand, considering the huge number of unnecessary tests and surgeries that are performed in the United States each year, I have to recognize that the principle behind managed care makes sense—at least as it pertains to knees. The problem comes with the implementation of this principle.

At the present, attempts at "managing" knee pain represent an enormous waste of time, energy, and money. The reasons for this are manifold.

TESTS

The tests that insurance companies want to manage are the particularly expensive and common tests, such as the MRIs (see chapter 2). However, approvals for such tests are carried out over the phone. Let us say your doctor wishes you to have an MRI. The insurance representative goes through a checklist that goes something like this:

• "Has the patient had X rays yet?" (This question is reasonable because, when carried out appropriately, X rays often give you all the information you need; see chapter 8). Your doctor's secretary indicates that X rays are negative.

• "Has the patient had any treatment?" "Yes, he had physical therapy."

• "What is the doctor looking for on the MRI?" "A torn meniscus" (cartilage). Based on this information, the MRI is approved.

At first glance, this seems sensible. It is not. The insurance company doesn't know that the X rays were probably inadequate. Of course, this can be the company's fault. They sometimes pay for just two X rays. Moreover, the insurance company doesn't know to what extent the physical therapy was adequate. Many therapy "factories" simply waste a person's time. Finally, and most significantly, it is not possible for the insurance company to know whether the doctor's examination was thorough enough to detect the many conditions that can be diagnosed without an MRI.

SURGERY

Approval for a surgical arthroscopy is addressed in a similar fashion. In addition to the above questions, the insurance representative will ask what the MRI showed. As noted in the previous chapters, regardless of what is truly wrong with you, the MRI report will often read "torn meniscus." This leads to an approval. And *voilà!* Despite inadequate evaluation and treatment, you and your doctor have just received approval for thousands of dollars' worth of tests and surgery.

Only education of the parties involved will eventually correct this problem.

MEDICATIONS

Prescription drugs represent a major portion of an insurance company's expenses, and it is understandable that the company would seek control over such costs. Once again, though, the devil is in the details. A number of companies function in a manner which is un-smart. For example, some plans charge patients a nominal flat fee for every prescription and will allow up to a three-month supply on any single prescription. Needless to say, patients subscribing to such plans will ask the doctor for a three-month supply of any medication at the very first office visit. To the patient this is three times less expensive than three one-month prescriptions. This is a reasonable policy for medications that are well known and well tolerated by the patient and must be taken for extended periods of time (e.g., blood-pressure medication). It is not reasonable for medications that a patient has never tried. Patients with knee pain sometimes have to test a few medications before they find the right one. Ordering three-month supplies of pills that will be discarded after two days' use is an enormous waste of resources. It is logical, then, to give the patient two prescriptions: one for a ten-day trial, and another for three months. Fat chance. The last thing the doctor wants to do is get into an economic discussion with a patient just because of some insurance policy. It would seem that most of the time the doctor writes the darned three-month prescription, and everybody pays the price. The first refill should be free.

And what about patients who get better after two to three weeks? They now have over two months of potentially expensive medications living in their medicine cabinet. As one can see, encouraging patients to order three-month supplies of pain medications on a routine basis is ludicrous.

But things get sillier. Some insurance companies will not cover inexpensive anti-inflammatory medications (NSAIDs). For example, one insurance company has recently stopped covering naproxen, which happens to be one of the time-honored NSAIDs. This same insurance company will, however, cover much more expensive NSAIDs that are neither better nor worse than naproxen. A phone call to the company led to the following comment: "We don't cover naproxen prescriptions because naproxen is available over the counter." As with many insurance rules, this would appear on the surface to make good sense. But any practicing knee doctor will tell you that this policy is flawed for at least two reasons: First, in a number of stores, naproxen is only available over the counter as Aleve. Aleve tablets are just under half the strength of the standard prescription (220 milligrams versus 500 milligrams), and you therefore have to take double the recommended dose (four tablets a day instead of two) to approach the prescription strength. At this dose, this brand medication Aleve is expensive compared to the generic prescription the insurance won't cover. The insurance company is therefore making you pay a lot for a drug that they can get for very little. Now there's a company with your interests in mind! Secondly, any doctor who's been in practice more than a week understands the importance of handing a prescription to a patient. Writing a prescription for naproxen is much more powerful than telling a patient to go buy Aleve. The doctor might as well say, "Take two aspirins and call me in the morning."[1] In short, because of shortsighted cost-cutting rules, doctors are driven to order expensive medications that end up costing insurance companies more money.

WORK INJURIES AND CAR ACCIDENTS

If you've been injured at work or in an automobile accident, your medical insurance shifts to Workers' Compensation or to your automobile insurance. In these instances, the insurance companies will try to control costs by having you see one of "their" doctors. For motor-vehicle accidents, no approval is needed for an MRI. Therefore, if you go to the right (wrong) doctor, you will as a matter of routine automatically be told to get an MRI of every part of your body that is remotely achy. This includes your knee, of course. If your doctor decides that you need surgery, the insurance company will send you for an IME (independent medical examination). Unfortunately, the "I" in IME is in the eye of the beholder! The insurance doctor is in fact paid to say that his insurance company is not responsible for the costs of your care. From my observation, I can tell you that an insurance company does not often rehire a doctor

---

1. In theory, doctors can sidestep this whole naproxen issue by prescribing one of the generic NSAIDs that is unavailable over the counter. But that's not the point. The whole business of remembering which insurance company covers which generic drug is very confusing.

who is truly fair and occasionally sides with the patient. Moreover, the insurance doctor will probably spend even less time examining you than your own doctor did, though that doesn't stop him from generating a three-page report. Finally, the insurance doctor sometimes isn't even asked to examine you until after the surgery!

If you've been injured at work, no significant test or treatment gets approved until you've seen a company doctor. This certainly makes more sense than being examined after the MRI and the surgery, but the system still does not work. It takes forever for an injured worker to be evaluated. It's as if the insurance company were thinking that by stalling the problem will go away. Mind you, this is often true, but it is not a healthy way to render health care. Many conditions will not simply go away, and some conditions actually are made worse by a delay.

Alas, in Workers' Compensation situations "the squeaky wheel gets the oil." It doesn't pay to sit tight and wait for things to happen unless you're in no particular hurry to get better and go back to work. Without being obnoxious, it pays to be persistent. Every doctor's office has dozens of patients waiting for approvals and company examinations and therefore cannot be counted on to apply steady pressure on the insurance companies. Consequently, it helps for patients to be their own advocates or to hire a lawyer.

Chapter 13

The Game

This world is a comedy to those that think, a tragedy to those that feel.

—Horace Walpole, "Letters"

I used to be disgusted, now I just try to be amused.

—E. Costello, "(The Angels Wanna Wear My) Red Shoes"

YOUR KNEE HURTS AS A RESULT OF AN INJURY, AND YOU'VE hired a personal-injury lawyer. Welcome to the "Game."

The Game features a code of ethics that may be different from what you are used to. Unless they are more honest than average, your experts and lawyers will be tempted to exaggerate your pain and disability. The insurance company, in my experience, can be expected to hire an "expert," who always sides with the insurance company. He will invariably state that there is nothing wrong with you that was not present before the accident. If you decide to quit in the middle of the Game or even just before the denouement, you can get paid for doing so! It's a dishonest game, and one hopes that this will change as lawyers and "experts" become better educated.

YOUR SIDE

No one but you knows just how much pain you're in, how much pain you had before the injury, and just how disabled you really are. If you go to a busy, honest lawyer, he or she will try to find out the truth and will tell you what your odds are of being compensated. A lawyer who is not busy and/or somewhat dishonest works differently.

I am constantly amazed by the number of injured parties who see a lawyer before seeing a doctor. This plays into the lawyer's hands. The somewhat unscrupulous lawyer sends his client to three equally unscrupulous doctors: a radiologist, who will automatically find a "torn cartilage" or ligament; an orthopedist who will gladly operate on this fictitious injury; and a rehabilitation doctor or chiropractor, who will provide months of treatment to back up your claim of severe pain and disability.

If, even before the accident, you were suffering from a condition that predisposed you to knee pain, the law is on your side. The law "takes you as you are." If you had a painless knee that was "an accident waiting to happen" and you sustain a tiny injury that sets off the pain, that tiny injury is responsible for all of your pain.

> In the eyes of the law, an accident is responsible for your pain even if you had a predisposition to pain.

In the eyes of the law, it is not the predisposing condition, but the injury that is responsible. If, metaphorically speaking, you carry a keg of gunpowder on your back, the spark that sets off the explosion is at fault. Let us assume, then, that you had a true torn cartilage before your accident. Let us further assume that this tear was painless. (This happens; see chapter 3.) If you are involved in an accident and your tear suddenly becomes painful, the accident is legally responsible for your pain.

The pain that you feel within the first few months of the injury is obviously important, but the potential long-term pain and disability should also be a concern to both you and your lawyer. Some injuries can continue to cause harm many years after the accident. For instance, the ends of your bone are lined with a thin layer of smooth, slippery cartilage called "articular cartilage." A diseased area of articular cartilage is called a chondral lesion (*chondro* means cartilage). If the cartilage is sufficiently damaged, painful arthritis can ensue. Initially, this damage may be visible neither to the naked eye nor on an MRI! In fact, even damage that is quite visible to the naked eye escapes detection on most MRIs!

The average lawyer doesn't know this. Instead, he or she will focus obsessively on the "torn cartilage" found by the radiologist. The plan is to show that your injury was severe enough to warrant surgery and months of therapy. In my opinion, this is a shortsighted plan. The torn cartilage is usually a figment of the radiologist's (well-paid) imagination. You cannot tear a cartilage by striking your knee against the ground or against a dashboard, and a small torn cartilage carries no long-term risks.

> The focus is too often on the nonexistent or insignificant "torn meniscus."

Why do lawyers continue to pursue this approach? Foremost, because they don't know any better. Moreover, sometimes it is better to go for the sure single than to try for the risky home run. Insurance companies have historically paid out settlements for torn cartilage without much of a fuss!

There are serious knee conditions that are not painful until the knee is traumatized. Kneecap malalignment is one of them. In some people, the kneecap (called the patella) doesn't sit right (see chapter 6). It is not necessarily a painful condition; in fact, many people live very well with it. This is particularly true of people who avoid jumping/twisting/bending activities. Trauma to the kneecap, however, triggers the malalignment pain. Thus, patients who land hard on their kneecap or strike their kneecap against a hard object suffer two types of pain at once: the pain from the contusion itself and the pain from the malalignment. This is a 1 + 1 = 3 situation in which the total is greater than the sum of the parts. I have dubbed it the "double crush" syndrome.[1] The existence of this double-crush syndrome explains why some people with apparently simple contusions continue to have pain long after it should have subsided. Patella malalignment can be a very difficult condition to treat, far more difficult than a little torn meniscus.

A common ploy of insurance companies is to state that a patient's kneecap malalignment was preexisting. To do so, they utilize a radiologist who will state that there are no signs of a fresh injury. This is disingenuous, since the MRI cannot always detect signs of fresh injury and certainly cannot tell what hurts.

Imagine a child growing up in a house by a cliff. As the child is playing in the garden, someone comes out of the bushes and pushes the child off the cliff. Whose fault is it that the child fell off the cliff? Is it the child's fault for living so close to the cliff,

---

1. I have borrowed the term from colleagues specializing in arm pain. The term *double crush* was originally used to describe a combination of a pinched nerve in the neck and a carpal tunnel syndrome in the hand, both of which can contribute to pain in the hand.

or is it the fault of the person who pushed the child? Although the child, through no fault of its own, was clearly at risk by being close to the cliff, the fault without doubt lies with the person doing the pushing. Likewise, a person with a poorly aligned kneecap is clearly at risk for developing pain, but the party at fault is the one who has traumatized the knee.

Three other conditions discussed in chapters 6 and 7 can be triggered by trauma: neuromas, tightness of the ITB (iliotibial band), and RSD (reflex sympathetic dystrophy). The experts on both sides routinely miss these. Meanwhile, patients are subjected to the unnecessary MRI, the unnecessary and unhelpful surgical arthroscopy, etc. If you've not done so already, read chapters 6 and 7 to see how you can tell if you've been checked for those conditions.

> RSD and neuromas are just some of the painful conditions that will not show up on an MRI!

THEIR SIDE

Once upon a time, I felt sorry for insurance companies and the people who pay their premiums (me, for example). I saw people trying to cash in on the slightest injuries, and it made my blood boil. The line between good and bad guys was clearly drawn. Now I see three camps: the insurance companies, the bad-guy plaintiffs (wanting huge awards for inconsequential injuries), and the good-guy plaintiffs (people truly wronged who deserve compensation).

> Insurance companies have seen so many cheats that they automatically assume you're one of them.

Without knowing anything about you, the insurance companies often treat you right off the bat as though you are one of the "bad guys." Admittedly, they have probably seen their fair share of cheats. They pay doctors to say that there is nothing wrong with you. Or if they can't dispute the existence of the condition, they say it was unrelated to the accident. Automatically. And that is the problem. The doctors are not simply exercising their constitutional right to voice an opinion. By routinely and automatically stating the same opinion over and over without regard for the merits of the case, these doctors are perjuring themselves for a fee. And doctors who refuse to play along aren't invited to play the game anymore.

> Doctors have made up their mind even before meeting you. They get away with this by hiding behind their right to an opinion.

If you've ever been subjected to this kind of insurance physical, you know that these doctors sometimes perjure themselves a second way: They do not even examine you! I recently treated a patient who, in addition to his knee condition, had a stiff, withered shoulder from a war injury. The insurance doctor had noted in his report "normal appearance of the shoulder" and had listed all its "normal" motions and functions! He hadn't even bothered to remove the patient's jacket.

This is partially the insurance companies' fault. They demand long-winded reports from doctors barely knowledgeable and uninterested in the part of the body that bothers you, let alone the rest of you. Whenever I've sent a succinct report stating my findings and opinion, it has been sent back with a request to "add a little more." So the doctors' secretaries bang out canned reports that may have no connection to reality. From having simply placed his hand on your knee, the doctor is able to produce a page filled with knee tests and, if pressed for time, may even be able to print out a complete neurological examination. This subterfuge is of no concern to the insurance companies so long as the doctors are not caught. Barring that very rare occurrence, insurance companies hide behind their doctors' right to a "medical opinion."

THE SETTLEMENT

Suppose you signed up for a million-dollar winner-take-all tournament. Now imagine being paid one hundred thousand dollars to drop out ("settle"). The great American tradition of the settlement is what makes the whole Game worthwhile. You don't have to win. You don't even have to be in the right. You just have to get the insurance companies to believe that you might win a jury over. Then they pay you to go away. For people who have truly been wronged, it is a fair system. For those who are dishonest, it is an easy scam.

> The great American settlement makes the whole Game worthwhile.

In summary, our current system is terribly unfair. Good and

bad guys are thrown into a lottery in which payouts appear to be randomly assigned. A minimal injury can win you a good settlement, yet the so-called experts often miss a serious injury, leaving you with no compensation. In a society that prides itself on fair play, it is surprising to me that such a system could still exist. I would favor an arbitration system whereby a panel of truly knowledgeable experts—not hired by either side—would pass judgment on the merits of knee injuries.

If your knee has truly been injured, and you have significant pain, your best bet is to consult an orthopedist who really understands your knee. Be prepared to be told the truth.

Chapter 14

On Bended Knee—The Future

MEDICINE, ORTHOPEDICS, AND SPECIFICALLY OUR UNDER-standing of knee problems have vastly increased during the last century. Our ability to treat knee conditions has improved to a staggering degree. Nevertheless, there is still a long road to travel before every person with knee pain can be successfully treated. In the first place, existing knowledge has to be more completely disseminated. The information presented in this book is not classified information buried in a top-secret Pentagon vault. It is widely available in textbooks and journals throughout the world. Yet most health professionals in the United States are not familiar with this information, a reflection of the huge amount of medical information currently available. There is so much in-formation that no single health professional can grasp it all. Even a well-trained orthopedic surgeon cannot absorb every-thing there is to know about orthopedic surgery. That is how large the field has become.

> If it does not concern erectile dysfunction, the diffusion of medical knowledge can be a maddeningly slow process.

The subtleties of the knee MRI and kneecap problems lie beyond the range of most health professionals dealing with the knee. They could learn it, of course. The material is not that complicated. It is simply missing from the textbooks and courses that most health professionals learn from.

If it does not concern erectile dysfunction, the diffusion of medical knowledge can be a maddeningly slow process.

Even more challenging are the conditions for which we do not even have a name, let alone a cure. Suppose you lived a hundred years ago and came down with lupus, a rheumatological condition that affects joints and organ systems. The doctors would have been unable to give you a diagnosis and incapable of discussing your condition with you. Had they cured you, it would have been strictly through luck. Because of the tremendous progress made in medicine over the last century, we have gradually come to believe that for every symptom there has to be a specific diagnosis that any competent doctor should be able to identify. Not so. Occasionally, people with (knee) pain suffer from conditions for which we have no name, no specific understanding, and therefore no precise treatment. Clearly, then, the medical profession must continue to investigate these mysterious conditions. Having said this, before you throw in the towel and assume that you are one of these unlucky people, make sure you see a knee specialist capable of detecting some of the oft-missed conditions listed in chapters 6 and 7.

> More accurate treatment and more reasonable insurance settlements can come only through education of doctors, lawyers, and judges.

On the legal and insurance front, much work needs to be done to assure fair reimbursements and compensation. The key is education. The insurance and legal "experts" must be trained to the point where they can legitimately call themselves expert. Right now, any orthopedist or rehabilitation specialist can call himself (or herself) an expert on the knee. This is nonsense. As we noted above, no orthopedist can know it all. Finally, lawyers and judges themselves need to be educated.

At the present, lawyers play tug-of-war over MRI reports they do not understand. In court, judges sustain or overrule questions pertaining to MRIs without themselves comprehending the limitations of these sophisticated tests.

The word *tear* (as in "tear of the cartilage") appears on a report, and it is assumed that the patient's problem has been ascertained. As we have discussed in the preceding chapters, an MRI does not indicate what hurts, an MRI cannot always differentiate between old and new, an MRI often shows a torn cartilage (meniscus) in patients without the least meniscal problem, and an MRI does not detect every single painful condition.

I look forward to the day when bogus tears of the meniscus "proven" by MRI are no longer compensated with five or more figures and when patients with long-lasting pain from difficult-to-treat conditions will no longer be accused of malingering. The faster we can educate the legal profession, the sooner we can rectify these unjust situations.

Chapter 15

How to Find the Right
Knee Doctor

AT THIS POINT, YOU'LL WANT TO FIND A DOCTOR WHO POS-
sesses the knowledge (and ethics) described in this book. For
this, you might consult:

1. the doctor nearest you
2. the doctor with the biggest ad in the phone book or the
   most impressive web site
3. the doctor recommended by your lawyer
4. the doctor referred by a friend or coworker
5. the team doctor for your favorite professional team
6. the doctor referred by your family physician
7. a doctor taken from the list of board-certified MDs, provided by a state medical society or by the American Acad-
   emy of Orthopaedic Surgeons

8. the doctor recommended by a hospital's referral service
9. a doctor listed in *The Best Doctors in (Your City)*
10. a doctor referred by a sports-medicine (nonsurgical) specialist
11. a doctor referred by a nurse, resident in training, or administrator at a hospital
12. a doctor with an impressive résumé
13. a department chairman
14. a doctor referred by another orthopedist

Each of these has merit, yet one stands out as being better than all others. Let us look at each individually:

The Doctor Nearest You

Obviously, by simply going to the doctor nearest you, you are taking a major gamble that requires no explanation.

The Doctor with the Biggest Ad in the Phone Book or the Most Impressive Web Site

Most savvy customers will know not to be impressed by an advertisement in the phone book. A large ad merely reflects the doctor's willingness to spend money on promotion, which is often effective, since most of the population are not savvy. Educated customers, though, can still be taken in by Web-page promotions. It is important to keep in mind that a doctor can make any claim on his or her home page. A health professional can pay to have an entire textbook on the Web! It doesn't mean that the health professional actually knows everything in that book or has even read it! The Web is merely the phone book of the new millennium.

The Doctor Recommended by Your Lawyer

As stated in an earlier chapter, a surprising number of Americans with knee pain see the doctor chosen by their lawyer. Although this is sometimes reasonable, very often the lawyer has a none-too-altruistic ulterior motive: dollars. Personal-injury lawyers who are not completely aboveboard know which radiologists will find something wrong on the MRI and which orthopedists will detect a condition that can be corrected only with months of therapy or surgery. Therefore, if there's nothing really wrong with you and you want to make some money, this is indeed the path to follow. Otherwise, beware.

The Doctor Referred by a Friend or Coworker

A doctor recommendation from a friend, relative, or coworker is fairly frequent. Everybody goes to the best doctor in town (ever hear of anybody going to the second best doctor around?), and people freely dispense advice. Such a recommendation tells you that at least someone has gotten better under that doctor's care—but it doesn't tell you if it was thanks to or in spite of the doctor. It also doesn't tell you about the doctor's ethics or knowledge of your particular problem. A guy who was great at treating your buddy's back pain may not be so hot when it comes to diagnosing your knee condition.

The Team Doctor for Your Favorite Professional Team

There's a reason why hospitals will pay professional teams a million dollars and up to have one of their docs be the team orthopedist: Being a team doctor is a terrific draw. And no book that anybody writes is going to change this. The thinking among the public is that "if he's good enough for the Jersey Jupiters, he's good enough for me." Having said this, is he good enough for the Jupiters? Usually yes, sometimes no. There are some very knowledgeable and ethical team doctors and some who are less so. The position of team doctor is not always won on merit.

The Doctor Referred by Your Family Physician

One thing that can be said for your family physician is that he or she has your best interests in mind—which is a start. Not all family physicians, though, recognize the intricacies of orthopedics to the point of differentiating between orthopedists who are particularly strong in one area versus those who are strong in another. Ask your doctor whether he or she would recommend the same orthopedist whether you had back or knee pain.

A Doctor Taken from the List of Board-Certified MDs, Provided by a State Medical Society or by the American Academy of Orthopedic Surgeons

Board certification is not a bad thing. If an orthopedist has been certified at some point by the American Board of Orthopedic Surgeons, it tells the potential customer that the surgeon has trained in an accredited American program and that he or she has studied hard to pass a written and oral examination. But in the setting of knee pain, board certification is not as important as it might seem. The board-certification examination covers an enormously wide range of subjects, including dwarfism, metallurgy, muscle physiology, cartilage biochemistry, wheelchair principles, and prosthetic limbs. Thrown in there are a few broad questions on knees.

Moreover, board certification is no guarantee of honesty, and as we have seen, it is very easy for an orthopedist to pull the wool over someone's eyes. In short, board certification is not a good selection criterion.

The Doctor Recommended by a Hospital's Referral Service

All major hospitals have a referral service, usually with a catchy toll-free telephone number, such as 1-877-COM TO US. They will never tell you, "We don't have anyone who does knees." Instead, they'll read you the names of orthopedists who have listed themselves as being interested in knees (or sports medicine or joint reconstruction). This, if you will, is the Yellow Pages of the hospital and just about as useful. You are better off contacting the orthopedic department directly, though here the staff will have some allegiance to the chairman and to his or her inner circle.

A Doctor Listed in *The Best Doctors in (Your City)*

There are a number of books purporting to give you a list of the best professionals around. Some are for real, and some are bogus. Here's how the bogus ones work: Doctors are sent an application to fill out: name, address, specialty, etc. The doctors who take the time to complete the form are included in the directory. When the book comes out, who buys it? All the doctors listed, of course! Everybody wins. The doctors are listed in a prestigious-sounding text, the publishing company earns a profit from all the doctors who bought the book, and nobody can accuse the doctors of having paid to be listed. Well, almost everybody wins. Anybody leafing through such a book in search of "the best doctors" is rolling the dice.

Other directories make more of an effort to truly find the best doctors. Be aware that they are imperfect, too. Some excellent surgeons toil in relative obscurity. They may not publish or lecture much and therefore will remain unknown outside their hospital. Others will have recently moved to a new hospital and not have formed a "base" yet. Yet others are of the shy, retiring type and will not attract any attention. This is somewhat rare for orthopedic surgeons. Read the first pages of any *Best Doctor* book to see how the doctors were selected.

A Doctor Referred by a Sports-Medicine (Nonsurgical) Specialist

A specialty has recently emerged called sports medicine, which is very confusing, because a number of medical and surgical specialties like to give themselves this title. The sports medicine I am referring to here is a medical (nonsurgical) specialty dealing with every aspect of athletic medicine, including injury, training, physiology, performance enhancement, management of concomitant medical conditions, etc. In the United States, there are still relatively few such doctors, and their prevalence varies considerably from state to state. They see and treat patients with knee pain and are therefore subject to the same issues discussed in the other chapters of this book. In other words, their understanding of the knee may or may not be limited. Nevertheless, since they do not operate, they usually have no personal interest in recommending unnecessary surgery, and when they refer a patient for surgery, it is likely to be to a good knee surgeon.

A Doctor Referred by a Nurse, Resident in Training, or Administrator at a Hospital

A hospital staff sees knee surgeons up close and personal. But few staff members see all the important aspects of a surgeon's practice. Nurses in the operating room get a sense of a surgeon's technical ability but can't say much about bedside manner or a surgeon's indications for surgery. Floor nurses can tell you about bedside manner and postoperative attention to patients but are less informed about technical ability and, again, surgical indications. Administrators can tell you which surgeons are busy but can't tell you why they are busy. (Are they good doctors or just good salesmen?) Residents (surgeons in training) are a good source of information with regard to the surgeons at their particular hospital, especially if they have a chance to participate in that surgeon's office hours. Because they are in training, though, they may lack some perspective and are susceptible to being won over by charismatic surgeons and/or swell guys who let them do cases. They also lack the ability to compare their teachers to other surgeons in town.

A Doctor with an Impressive Résumé

An impressive résumé tells you that the surgeon has given a great deal of thought to an area of study. If he is asked to lecture, he is probably thought of as being knowledgeable, and more significantly, if he has been widely published, he probably has expertise in the area of his publications. A résumé, though, doesn't tell you about patient management and ethics.

A Department Chairman

The chairman of an orthopedic department is suave, debonair, good-looking, intelligent, and highly skilled,[1] and it is natural for patients to seek out the advice of such a doctor. Chairmen (chairwomen are quite rare, perhaps nonexistent in orthopedics) are chosen on the basis of their particular expertise in one area

1. My chairman could conceivably be reading this book.

of orthopedics and/or leadership and administrative skills. Their appreciation of the subtleties of the knee ranges from excellent to minimal, depending on their area of expertise. Chairmen are usually surrounded by a well-organized staff and have the full attention of senior orthopedic residents (residents in their last year of training). This may or may not compensate for the fact that some chairmen are away from their practice a great deal. Make sure this is not something that would bother you.

A Doctor Referred by Another Orthopedist

Bingo. A referral from an orthopedist is not easy to come by unless you happen to be related to one or have one as a friend. (Everybody should!) Nevertheless, this is your best bet. You might even consider paying for a consultation just to get such a referral. Orthopedists know the orthopedic BSers in their community as well as the guys with suspect ethics better than any layperson and, for obvious reasons, better than doctors in other specialties. The advice of an orthopedist is not foolproof, of course. If you live in a large community, no orthopedist will be familiar with the particular strengths and shortcomings of all his colleagues. If the orthopedist has something bad to say about the doctor you had in mind, it could be because of rivalries and jealousies. Conversely, an orthopedist may be interested in helping a friend. Nevertheless, it is unlikely that an orthopedist would let you make a big mistake.

In an ideal world, you would have access to all of the above options, and they would all point to one or two knee doctors in your community. Realistically, you will have access to just a few of the options I have listed. My advice would be to use as many as possible.

Chapter 16

Answers to Common Questions (and to Those You Should Be Asking!)

What exactly is a torn cartilage?

Cartilage is the rubbery shock absorber that lies between the thighbone and the shinbone. In fact, there are two in each knee, one on the inside (medial) and one on the outside (lateral). The medical term for cartilage when used in this setting is meniscus. The back (posterior) aspect of the meniscus is the weakest. A common finding on the MRI is therefore "tear of the posterior horn of the medial meniscus." What you need to know is that most tears thus identified on an MRI are of *no clinical relevance* (see chapter 3).

What is "knee arthritis"?

There is another type of cartilage in the knee: that which lines the ends of the bones. (Look at the end of a chicken bone.)

This cartilage is called articular cartilage. When this cartilage wears down to bone, arthritis is said to have set in. Arthritis can be present in just one part of the knee or can be present throughout. Arthritis can coexist with a torn cartilage (meniscus), but it is a completely different entity.

What is a locked knee?

It's a knee that is stuck. It just won't straighten. A true locked knee is usually caused by a large tear of the meniscus, such as a "bucket handle" tear (see chapter 3). Most of the time, locking is really pseudolocking. The knee won't straighten or bend because it just hurts too much to do so. A little pain medication by mouth or a Novocain injection solves the problem. This type of pseudolocking is not indicative of a serious problem. You can get pseudolocking with a simple, plain, torn MCL (see chapter 4). True locking requires surgery, though it is *not* a medical emergency.

Is osteoarthritis the same as osteoporosis?

There is no connection between the two. The words sound somewhat the same because they start with "osteo," but that's where the similarity ends. Osteoarthritis is the most common type of arthritis, arthritis being the wearing out of articular cartilage (see above). Osteoporosis, on the other hand, is the thinning and weakening of bone and has nothing to do with cartilage. You can have osteoarthritis with or without osteoporosis and vice versa.

Everybody says I need an MRI. Is that true?

Probably *not*. The MRI is an extraordinary test. It is extremely accurate for tumors and fractures, and if this is what your doctor is looking for, then, yes, you should have an MRI. An MRI is also reasonably accurate for certain torn ligaments.

If you've had a major injury and the doctor suspects a tear of that ligament, then again, yes, an MRI is reasonable. There are also unusual conditions here and there that are best diagnosed with an MRI (see chapters 6 and 7). By and large, however, most knee MRIs are a waste of time. They are *not* terribly accurate for tears of the meniscus (torn cartilage) and even less so for subtle arthritis. There are MRI centers where every patient is said to have a torn cartilage. This finding on an MRI therefore has minimal value. More importantly, there are a number of painful conditions that are not detected on an MRI. Most significant of all, the MRI cannot tell the doctor what hurts! Not every tiny variation on an MRI is a source of pain! Even a nice sunny day can have a few little clouds.

Now that MRIs exist, should I even bother with X rays?

Yes. Despite what you might have heard, a good set of X rays provides the doctor with a great deal of information.

True or False? All X rays are pretty much the same.

False. Most X rays are too basic. The traditional set consists of two X rays taken with the patient lying down. Such X rays reveal major fractures and moderate-to-advanced arthritis. More sophisticated X rays are required to detect less advanced arthritis and kneecap problems. These sophisticated X rays are still far simpler and less expensive than an MRI.

What is the difference between a CT scan and a CAT scan?

None.

What is the difference between an MRI and CT (CAT) scan?

They both slice you up radiographically like a loaf of bread. The CT scan does so with X rays, and the MRI uses magnetic resonance that involves no radiation. CT is classically better for fine bony detail, and MR imaging is better for nonbony tissue, for example, cartilage and ligaments. A CT scan is currently less expensive. An MRI cannot be carried out on someone with a metallic implant that is magnetic.

What is a bone scan?

This also goes by the name *nuclear bone scan,* and it tests the "activity" of bone. Bone is a living tissue. Bone cells "turn over." They die and are replaced. In the bone-scan study, a slightly radioactive tracer is injected intravenously into the subject. The tracer hitchhikes onto all the bones in the body as they go about their daily business of replenishing themselves. In a bone that is more active than usual, more tracer will be picked up. When the subject is placed under a Geiger-counter type of device, that bone will appear "hot."

My knee makes funny noises. Is that a problem?

No, not if it doesn't hurt. There are many layers of tissue moving over and around the bones of the knee. If any of these tissues becomes a little thick, it will snap the way a rubber band might twang if it is stretched across the corner of a table. It is of no consequence.

What is chondromalacia?

A very confusing term meaning many things to many people. I would tell you to ignore it except that people still use it. There is still an insurance code for it. It can mean (1) pain in the front of the knee, (2) pain coming from the kneecap, (3) cartilage abnormalities under the kneecap, (4) articular cartilage abnormalities anywhere in the knee, or (5) articular cartilage abnormalities in any joint of the body!

Is it better to apply heat or cold to the knee?

You can apply heat or cold. Usually, if you've just hurt your knee, you should apply something cold, though not right on the skin. After two days, switch to heat. If your knee is chronically painful, heat usually works best. Some people feel best when they alternate between heat and cold. Try it (see chapters 3 and 5).

I've been told that I have torn cartilage. Do I need surgery?

There is about a 5 percent chance that this is true. Most of the torn cartilages are diagnosed on an MRI and do not represent real tears (see chapters 2 and 3). Of the tears that really exist, only a portion of those cause pain and require surgery.

True or False? I'm over sixty-five, I've had knee pain a long time, and my surgeon says an MRI would be a waste of time.

True. Your pain is likely to be mostly from arthritis. You don't need a weatherman to know which way the wind blows, and you don't need an MRI to tell someone over the age of sixty-five that their chronic pain is due to arthritis. A good X ray usually suffices (see chapter 8).

I'm forty years old, I like to bike, and I tore my ACL. Do I need surgery?

No. If you're over forty years old and your favorite activities don't involve twisting, you don't need to have your ACL reconstructed. If, however, your knee gives out even after adequate rehabilitation, you may indeed require surgery.

I'm having an ACL reconstruction. What is a "graft"?

The current thinking is that a torn ACL will not heal even if it is stitched back together. Tissue has to be taken from somewhere to create a new ligament from scratch. This new ligament is called a graft. It can come from a number of places around your knee, it can be procured from a tissue bank, and it can be made of a synthetic material. In the United States, synthetic grafts have not had a good track record.

I need a knee replacement. I'll search the Internet for the best new implant. Is this a good idea?

No. Surprisingly, most new implants fail within a few years. For the majority of patients, a knee replacement with a long track record is the best bet.

I need a knee replacement, but I'm scared. Am I wrong?

Yes and no. Complications can be disastrous, but they occur less than 1 percent of the time. If your pain is tolerable, this less than 1 percent is still too big a risk. But once that pain becomes severe and unrelenting, "less than 1 percent" should look pretty good.

I have a prescription for physical therapy. Does it matter where I go?

It depends on what exactly your condition is. For "routine" arthritis any good therapy center will be fine. On the other hand, if your pain stems from a kneecap problem, many exercises will actually aggravate your pain. In this situation, you must be in the hands of a therapist who really understands the kneecap and who will give you the attention you need.

An MRI should be able to tell me why my knee hurts, right?

Wrong. Go back to chapter 2. Can a computer tell you who's pretty? The MRI will reveal umpteen details of your knee but can't say what hurts. Your knee pain might not even be coming from the knee! Certain hip conditions are known to masquerade as knee pain. Don't be too quick to believe that the "abnormality" on the MRI is the source of your pain.

My insurance wants me to go for an independent medical examination. The doctor will examine me thoroughly and give an honest opinion, right?

Wrong. In my experience, many insurance doctors perform a perfunctory examination, print out long canned reports, and state that there is nothing wrong with you that wasn't there before. They hide behind the concept that they are entitled to their opinion (see chapter 12).

This pain medication is expensive! Why is that?

When a medication is released, it is patented by the parent company, the one that paid for the development of that medication. No one else can manufacture or sell this medication. The company can charge whatever it wants. This follows the basic laws of supply and demand. When the patent runs out, any company can start to sell the drug. Competition lowers the price. New drugs therefore cost more than older ones. New drugs are even sometimes better than older ones.

If I have arthritis, should I take calcium?

You should probably take calcium, but not because you have arthritis. Calcium controls osteoporosis, and osteoporosis is not related in any way to arthritis (see above).

Do nutritional supplements work?

Generally speaking, taking nutritional supplements is a good idea. Most people do not ingest the right mix of vitamins and minerals and should supplement their diet. Whether nutritional supplements help the pain of arthritis or of any other condition is still unknown. Figuring out whether a pain treatment is effective or not is more complicated than it seems (see chapters 5 and 9).

I hurt my knee, and I'm in agony. I'll probably need surgery. Right?

Not so fast. The pain of an injury can get you to sign just about any surgical consent. You can't believe you'll ever feel any better. And yet, no matter how bad the pain is, chances are it will improve dramatically over the next few days. Of course, in the end you may require surgery, but the initial pain is no indication of whether that will or will not come to pass.

Should I try a brace?

It doesn't hurt to try. Unless you have a tear of the MCL (see chapter 4), the beneficial effects of a brace are not predictable. They don't have side effects, so try one. Your doctor or therapist should be able to point you in the right direction.

Are injections really bad for you?

Steroid (cortisone) injections can damage tissues over time. Although they reduce inflammation and diminish pain, in time you may pay the price. Hyaluran and related products, on the other hand, are natural to the extent that they are found in the human knee to begin with. They are not as likely to be harmful but are also less likely to reduce acute pain.

INDEX

177